Christina Koller

# Breathe Consciously, Live Intensely

## VAGUS FLOW® – The Art of Breathing

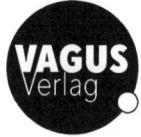

# Contents

# Part 2 · Exercises 84

# Foreword

In the course of our daily lives, we change our breathing rhythms unconsciously - again and again. Even back and forth, hectic or calm, prolonging or shortening life. At least always, otherwise we would no longer be here!

Our breath of life has been given a lot of attention in this book and it is worth rethinking how we deal with it.

It would be so important to (learn to) fill our own breath with much more awareness. This shows around and in our eyes, not just with a smile.

With my way of analysing the eyes and with the methods of the Polyvagal Theory (Stephen W. Porges), I always find my way back to the rhythm of the human breath in my working life. Expressly, when I am allowed to carry out an eye analysis. We humans can keep ourselves more tired or more active with the feedback mode of our own breath. Isn't that marvellous? It is the vagal circuits of our own breathing frequency that can unleash unexpected forces or brakes within us. Every breathing frequency allows us to draw important conclusions about our current health. Visible in the sclera and iris of both eyes. Right eye sympathetic / left eye parasympathetic / comparison of both eye differences shows the current vagus state.

Healthy people breathe passively - on average 10 to 15 times per minute. This respiratory volume is 6 to 9 litres of air per minute; around 0.5 litres per breath. This equates to around 23,000 breaths and around 12 cubic metres of air per day. An enormous power that can be utilised if we want to!

In this book, Christina Koller shows us so beautifully how we can learn to re-calibrate our own breathing - how life will flow more smoothly again if we integrate the many exercises she has provided.

Enjoy reading, slow down, simplify and deepen.

*Prof. Rita Fasel, Bürgenstock*
*www.ritafasel.ch*

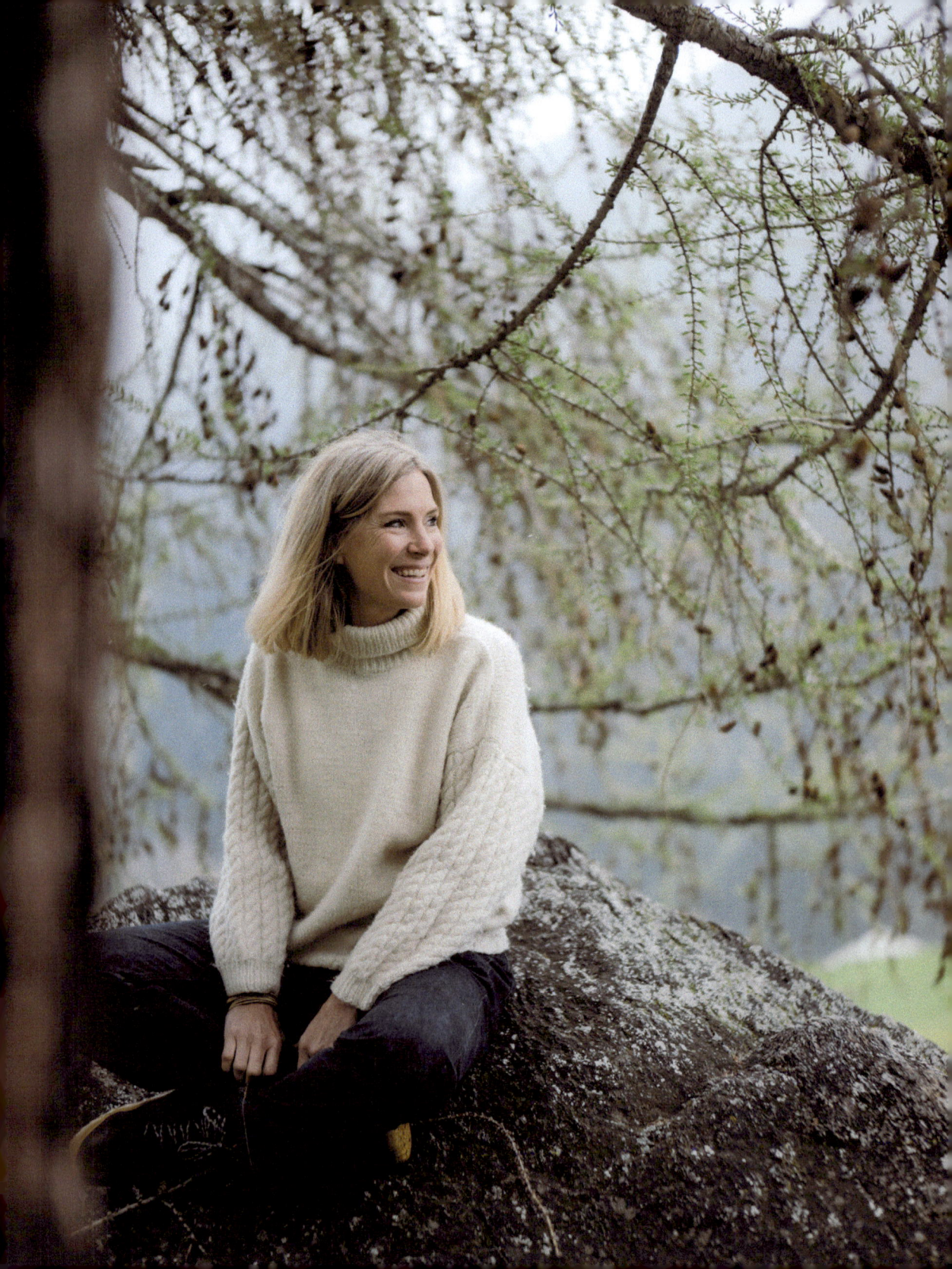

*I Dedicate this Book to*

*Till Akira*
*&*
*Luna Makena*

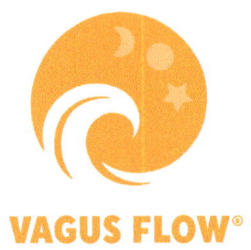

**VAGUS FLOW®**

„May VAGUS FLOW® give you the courage to face your deepest fears, pursue your highest dreams and live a life of authenticity and contentment."

# A Word at the Beginning

## *Dear Reader*

In an everyday life that often leaves us hardly any time to breathe, I invite you to welcome every moment with open arms and an alert heart with „Breathe consciously - live intensively" and the VAGUS FLOW® method. Your breath is your constant guide.

On my path, which has taken me through many years of in-depth training in social work, yoga and breathing therapy, I have gained deep insights into the human psyche, the body and its incredible ability to heal itself. I have completed each of these training programmes with a certificate, but the real certificate lies in the experiences and the changes I have been able to bring about in myself and others.

These insights and experiences lead to VAGUS FLOW®, a method that uses the power of your breath to harmonise you with yourself and the world around you.

The vagus nerve is a central player in your parasympathetic nervous system and is your key to deep relaxation and well-being.

**With VAGUS FLOW® you get:**

**Exercises Suitable for Everyday Life**
Discover how a few minutes of mindfulness every day can stimulate your vagus nerve and significantly improve your overall well-being.

**Strengthen your Emotional Resilience**
Recognise how you can reduce stress, reduce anxiety and increase your emotional resilience through conscious breathing.

**Improved Physical and Mental Health**
Experience the positive effects on the cardiovascular system, digestion and immune system.

**Deeper Self-Knowledge**
Find self-knowledge and self-love through the mindful connection of body and mind.

My method is designed to integrate seamlessly into your everyday life. No special equipment or extraordinary circumstances are required. Whether at the beginning of your day, during a short break at work or as a quiet finale in the evening - VAGUS FLOW® is your constant companion as you take steps towards a safer and more fulfilling life.

Through my developed concept, VAGUS FLOW®, you will learn to breathe consciously, to be connected with your emotions and thus to live more intensely.

The inner journey is the greatest life adventure that makes you rich and shows you how to recognise every day as a special gift.

SUSTAIN, SIMPLIFY, DEEPEN – these principles lead you back to your natural rhythm and into the now. Life becomes easier when you are present. This presence invites you to relax and deepen your experiences.

RECOGNISE: Patience, mindfulness and perseverance will be your companions on this journey. Sometimes the mind may be faster than the heart, but trust that both will come into harmony to support you.

I recommend taking notes to intensify your thoughts and realisations. These notes are not only a tool for your personal development, but also a space for reflection, insight and growth.

I look forward to sharing my experiences with you and accompanying you on the path to your inner strength. May VAGUS FLOW® give you the courage to shape your life in an authentic and fulfilling way.

*With best regards, Christina Koller*

# About Me

## „Slow Down, Simplify and Deepen."

At the age of 17, I left home to explore the world as a globetrotter. On my journey through life, I experienced highs and lows and gained valuable life experience.

After many hellish rides and low blows, I created the life that suits me from the depths. Harmful structures and behaviours, destructive people automatically lost access to me. Through this liberation, I was able to recompose and reorganise myself.

I now draw from the full and bring my experiences, combined with my expertise, to the outside world. I want to encourage and empower people to shed layer upon layer of their numbness and woundedness so that they can once again hear their very own rhythm, their heart's voice, their needs and their dreams.

Over the past three decades, I have expanded and explored my knowledge and experience in tourism, social work, yoga and breathing therapy.

Three concepts move me and I always put them centre stage:
**Slowing down, simplifying and deepening.**

As a breath therapist, I am passionate about my values. I apply them in all areas of my life and constantly check whether I am being true to myself.

The holistic fascinates me deeply, as does the power of communication and the refinement of the choice of words. My life has been characterised by an intense preoccupation with people.

In the majestic Engadine mountains, my home, I find peace, inspiration and strength. This is where I recharge my batteries and find myself again.

The births of my two children were the most powerful moments of my life. Spending time with them is invaluable to me and enriches my life in a way that can hardly be put into words.

I am deeply grateful for the variety and diversity that life has given me. I allow myself to savour all these opportunities, knowing where my roots and my happiness are at home.

My horses are my faithful companions, they make me laugh and keep me healthy. I experience the freedom and wildness of the Engadin most intensely on long gallops through the woods. Endless forays through thickets and mountains are just as much a part of me as picking berries, mushrooms and plants. Nature is my retreat and my source of inspiration.

Breathing, meditation and physical work have kept me fit and helped me to connect with myself.

I enjoy being alone, reading, travelling, dancing and writing. But I also value the dialogue and inspiration I find in the company of others.

## How it All Began

„There it was - that breath that changed my life.
A moment of the deepest disorientation and of darkness.
Nothing on the outside could give me stability and
support. And suddenly it flowed through me.
A quiet silver thread of hope and direction appeared
before me.
It was this one breath that healed my world and
reassembled me - resurrected me and breathed life
into me.
I felt my body. Trust in myself returned, guided
by the breath and a new confidence."

The moment I described, the one deep breath that changed my life, symbolises the vital power that lies in every single breath.

Our breathing is more than just an automatic process. It is a gateway to our inner self, a tool to regulate our emotions and a way to improve our wellbeing. Conscious breathing unites the heart and mind.

The aim is to support you on your personal journey and give you tools to use your breathing as a source of healing and personal transformation. Be invited to be open to new experiences and allow yourself to explore your breath and your inner world in order to write your personal story.

The illustrations are simplified schematic representations of anatomy and physiology. They are intended to help you understand the VAGUS FLOW® theory and its effect on the body and psyche.

*Have fun discovering and experiencing.*

Register and get free access to
the colour illustrations.

Illustrations at:
**www.sanajer.ch**

# My Mission

*Hey you, yes, exactly you!*
I am here to invite you on an exciting journey to your essence. As an experienced practitioner of the art of breathing and creator of the VAGUS FLOW® method, I am here to be your personal guide. Together we will awaken the courage within you to not only exist, but to shine and realise your full potential.
I am here to encourage you to not only recognise your uniqueness, but to live it!

**Why the Breath?**
Ah, the breath! So simple, so clear, so honest.
Imagine holding a magic wand in your hand - that's your breath. It connects your body with your mind and chats non-stop with your autonomic nervous system. Every breath is a step on the path to you.
Your breath never lies - it is your personal compass that supports and guides you always and everywhere.

*Jump with me into a life full of awareness, energy and natural, fulfilling breaths. With VAGUS FLOW®, this is no longer a dream – it's your new reality.*

**What you get from me and VAGUS FLOW®**

**Experience**
I give you my extensive knowledge from around 25 years of work experience in accompanying and guiding people, the practice and teaching of yoga and breathing therapy, which I have gathered in my own centre.

**Breath Awareness**
Let me show you how you can let your breath awareness flow naturally into your everyday life. Inhale the essence of the world of breath with me.

**Knowledge that Inspires**
Discover the secrets of breath, vagus nerve, nervous system and more - everything you need to understand and harmonise yourself and your emotions.

**Practical Magic**
I don't just give you theory, I equip you with real, life-changing and mind-opening practices.

**Your Toolbox**
Strengthen your breath awareness and body awareness with methods specifically designed to peel the onion and make you shine.

**Emotional Navigator**
Learn to recognise your emotions and to allow, endure, embrace and integrate them.

**Goodbye Stress!**
I'll show you how to break the stress cycle and catapult yourself into a state of calm and regeneration or into healthy activity.

**Live your Dream**
Together we will pave the way for you to live your dreams and achieve your goals with joy.

# Part 1 · Theory

In this chapter, we look at basic theories around breathing, the autonomic nervous system (ANS) and the vagus nerve. Our aim is to slow down, simplify and deepen these complex topics so that you can develop a sound understanding of the connections between breathing and the regulation of the ANS and the vagus nerve.

Breathing is a vital function of our body that is often automatic but can also be consciously controlled. In this chapter, we will explore how your breathing not only brings oxygen to your body, but also influences your mood and quality of life.

The vagus nerve, also known as the ‚wandering nerve', plays a crucial role in regulating various bodily functions, including heart rate, digestion and inflammatory responses. We will look at how purposefully slowing and deepening your breathing can help to promote the activation of your vagus nerve, thereby reducing stress, promoting relaxation and harmony.

By exploring various theoretical topics and the VAGUS FLOW® concept, we lay the foundation for understanding and applying the practical breathing techniques that we will explore later in the book.

## „Breath – physical life begins with the first inhalation and ends with the last exhalation."

# Facts and Figures About Breathing

Breathing is an inconspicuous act, but it has an immense effect on our body and our biochemistry. To understand why breathing deserves so much attention, let these figures sink in:

· The nose filters every breath (during nasal breathing). When you breathe in, it warms the air and filters out around 100,000 bacteria and 200,000 viruses. When you breathe out, it retains moisture in the body. This is one of the reasons why nasal breathing is so important.

· Our outer skin has an area of 2 square metres, the lungs cover around 70 square metres and the intestines 250 to 400 square metres.

· If the oxygen supply is cut off, we are brain dead within 30 seconds.

· We excrete 70% of toxins via exhalation, 20% via the skin, 7% via the bladder and 3% via the intestines. In stress mode, exhalation and thus the elimination of toxins is reduced.

· At rest, an adult breathes in 0.5 litres of air; conscious breathing takes in 2 to 5 litres. An asthmatic reaches up to approx. 15 litres (this is overbreathing and can lead to hyperventilation and even fainting).

· The influence of breathing on the autonomic nervous system (ANS) is significant, as it is the only area of the ANS that we can control voluntarily. It can have both a calming and a stimulating effect.

· There is no right or wrong way to breathe. Your perception is always correct.

· Every breath provides oxygen, which our body needs to produce energy. Without a sufficient supply of oxygen, various organs and tissues cannot function properly.

· A healthy diet and lifestyle are of little help if stress breathing is our norm.

· Overbreathing is a condition in which we inhale more air than our body needs. Most people in our part of the world breathe too much and too quickly.

· Through targeted breathing techniques, we can reduce stress, increase concentration and recognise our emotions. Regulation to the desired state becomes possible. This illustrates the close connection between our breathing and our mental well-being.

**To Summarise**

It is essential to breathe consciously and to ensure that we do not breathe unnecessarily quickly or deeply in order to avoid over-breathing and to maintain our body's biochemical balance. We should definitely practise nasal breathing, as this is the prerequisite for healthy, natural breathing and its holistic influence on our health and well-being.

**Example**

A simple example illustrates the power of breathing: in stressful situations, we tend to breathe more shallowly and quickly. If we learn to do the exact opposite in such moments, namely to consciously deepen and slow down our breathing, we counteract the stress and put our body in a relaxed state.

*„The quality of our breathing determines the quality of our life."*

# Breath Therapy - Three Types of Breath

Breath therapy is a profound practice that goes beyond the simple application of breathing exercises and requires several years of training. Although the breathing techniques can be learnt relatively quickly, the real art lies in the emotional process: it is about establishing a connection to one's own emotions, allowing them and enduring them without following the immediate impulse to repress or change them.

This ability to look deep into one's own inner abysses and offer support to others requires not only solid basic psychological training, but also experience and the willingness to devote oneself regularly and with dedication to this process.

To better understand the complexity of breathwork, it is helpful to take a closer look at the following three terms:

## Unconscious

The majority of our breathing occurs unconsciously. Without us having to actively think about it, our breath supplies us with oxygen and thus enables us to live. This unconscious breathing automatically adapts to our physical needs, be it during sleep, physical exertion or rest. The breathing pattern reflects our thoughts and emotions and is constantly changing.

## Conscious

Conscious breathing means that we focus our attention on our breath. Through this conscious awareness and simply allowing what is going on inside us at the moment, the emotion changes automatically without our active intervention. Did you know that emotions change within 20 minutes if we allow them to do so completely? We can dedicate ourselves to meditation and relaxation by observing our breathing. Conscious breathing is a tool that helps us to be in contact with our body and our emotions. This promotes our resilience.

**Guided Breath**

Guided breath goes one step further and involves the intentional control of breathing rhythm, depth and technique. This type of breathing is often used in respiratory therapy to specifically influence certain physical or emotional states. It requires knowledge, practice and awareness and is a powerful tool to support healing processes in the body and mind.

Breath therapy combines these levels of breathing to promote a holistic sense of well-being and to accompany people on their individual journey through their own lows and highs.

*„With my method, I pave the way for the activation of the anterior vagus branch and its associated cranial nerves. Understanding and utilising these processes is the basis for a successful therapeutic experience.*

*My work includes not only conversations that touch the heart, but also massages that revitalise the body and breathing and physical exercises that nourish the soul.*

*Each session is an invitation to delve deeper into one's self, to awaken hidden powers and to harmonise body and mind.*

*Together we discover the healing power of the breath, which enables us to go through life with serenity and new energy."*

# The Philosophy of VAGUS FLOW®

**Breathe**

„Everything begins with a breath. Breathe out. Then the next breath. The breath connects our inside with the outside. This can be seen in physical terms, but it can also be seen in psychological terms. The breath connects our inner calm (or restlessness) with the challenges of the world in which we find ourselves. By breathing calmly, we can consciously create a moment of stillness, discover, find silence and connect with ourselves and the surrounding nature. In this way, we can discover new strength and find clarity.

Everyone has their own path in life and there is no right or wrong. It is not about reaching a certain goal, but about better understanding ourselves, our own way of being. On this journey of discovery, we learn many things and have experiences that help us to see the world, ourselves and our relationship to the world more clearly.

The most important thing is not even the learning itself, but how we apply what we have learnt in our lives, i.e. in other life situations. It is worth striving to get in touch with yourself, to feel and perceive your own inner truth.

An important question for me is: How well am I connected with myself? That is why I am increasingly focussing on what I feel myself, in addition to what others say. What counts is strengthening this connection to myself.

No anger or rejection should permanently destroy the inner peace and love within me. Deep down, I have always been strong, I have always been loved. Deep down, I am connected to everything. I also find you inside me.

It all began with a breath. And every further breath is a reminder of how important it is to be connected to yourself."

The exploration of the self and the universal search for deep love and understanding of our existence are the cornerstones of VAGUS FLOW®, a method that strives for harmony not through restrictions, but through the conscious experience and integration of all aspects of life. The core of this practice is the acceptance and flow of emotions, which promotes an authentic, awake and rooted being.

VAGUS FLOW® understands true insight and self-understanding as natural states of being. These are accessed through the acceptance and experiencing of emotions, a process that teaches us to embrace the full range of human experience.

This method emphasises that the answers we seek are not to be found in external sources, but in connecting with our inner self. By recognising and allowing our own light and full range of emotional being, we discover aliveness and authenticity.

Leaving the conventional spiritual quest behind, I have fully embraced VAGUS FLOW®, a path that emphasises the silent acceptance of our emotions and shows us how to live in harmony with our feelings. This journey has taught me that deep at my core, I am not only loved and untouched, but also dynamic and rich in emotional experiences - experiences that I share with all of humanity.

I have learnt to accept emotions as part of my experience and allow them to shift naturally, leading to true peace and understanding. This acceptance creates a space in which we recognise not only ourselves, but also our deep connection with others. It is a path that leads us to a deeper truth: We are all connected, in light, love and in the infinite dance of our emotions.

## The Breath as the Key

The core principles of VAGUS FLOW® - slowness, simplicity and depth - invite us to return to the essence of our existence - our breath. This is a guide to a more mindful lifestyle and a bridge to connecting with the universe:

### Slowness
reduces the hectic pace of everyday life and creates moments of pause and conscious breathing that offer us space for introspection.

### Simplicity
frees our lives from the superfluous and brings us back to the basic form of the breath, allowing us to discover beauty, joy and clarity.

### Depth
enables a more intense connection to our breath and thus to our essence, improves the quality of each breath and opens paths to inner peace.

The teaching guides you through a conscious practice characterised by ethics (values), self-care, body and breath awareness, sensory clarification, focus, meditation and union, always guided by the three pillars - slowness, simplicity and depth.

„The boundaries we feel in life are often only those that our thoughts erect. They keep us trapped in our own cage."

### Values

Start by reflecting on your behaviour and acting more consciously. This practice asks you to pause and consider the effects of your actions. We have often adopted values from our ancestors without reflection. We think that this value is important, but do not feel it.

### Self-care

Concentrate on getting to know yourself, look inwards and give yourself time and attention. In connection with the values, feel what you feel, what you are passionate about and what you stand for. Apply this in all areas of your life.

### Body awareness

Use movements to dive deeper into the connection with your body and become aware of your body.

### Breath - VAGUS FLOW® Breath Essence:

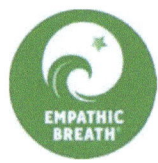

**Empathic Breath**

To strengthen the ventral vagal state, we train body awareness of feelings. This promotes empathy, resilience, joy and safety.

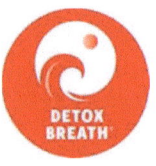

**Detox Breath**

We regulate the sympathetic state by using dynamic breathing and physical exercises to reduce stress and strengthen resilience.

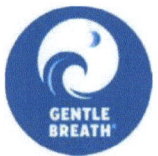

**Gentle Breath**

To find our way out of the dorsal vagal state, we use this form to gently and mindfully move out of rigid states and activate our healing powers.

The chosen colours of Empathic, Detox and Gentle Breath harmonise with those of the wave (page 43).

## Sensory Clearing

Withdraw from constant external stimulation and direct your attention inwards to clear and purify your senses. This will help you to return from a state of overstimulation to natural relaxation. It is extremely important to integrate body and breath awareness.

## Focussing

Slowing down your thoughts: By sifting out unnecessary thoughts and focussing on a single topic, you calm your mind, which marks the beginning of deepening into stillness and peace.

## Meditation

Means immersion. Choose a topic or word of your choice and clarify your self-perception and the feelings associated with it. In meditation you will find peace and clarity through concentration.

## Union

Achieve depth, calm and the ultimate simplification of your being through union with yourself and the world around you.

VAGUS FLOW® is more than a method; it is a way of life that leads to a more intense connection with yourself and the world through unwinding and simplification. This journey back to your true self is guided by the simplicity and stillness of your breath and heart.

# Autonomous Nervous System

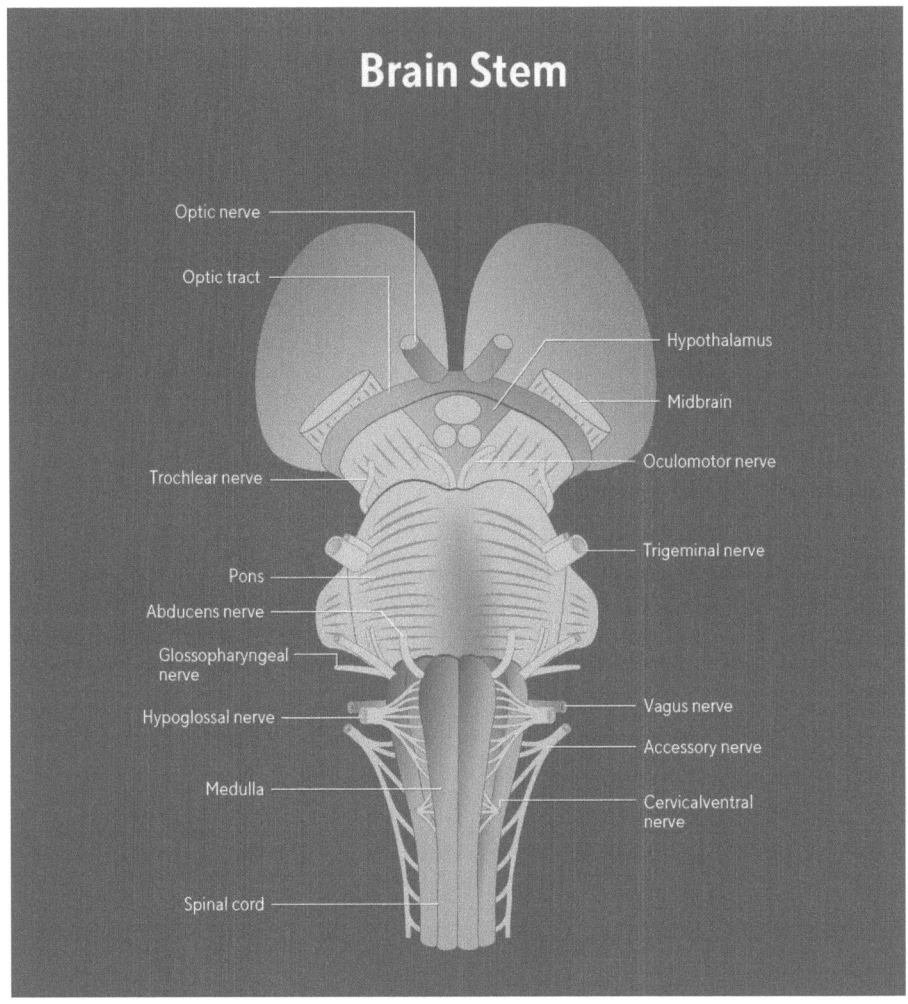

The autonomic nervous system (ANS) is the body's main control centre and regulates the organs, including the hormonal and respiratory systems. It controls all vital functions such as the cardiovascular system, respiration, blood pressure, digestion, immune system and reproduction.

„Chronic stress is a bio-chemical and neurophysiological rampage in the human organism and should be consistently combated."
Dr Siddhartha Popat, MD

Interestingly, breathing is the only area of the central nervous system that I can actively influence and control. By consciously influencing my breathing, I can actively control the ANS, communicate directly with my brain and escape the stress-exhaustion cycle.

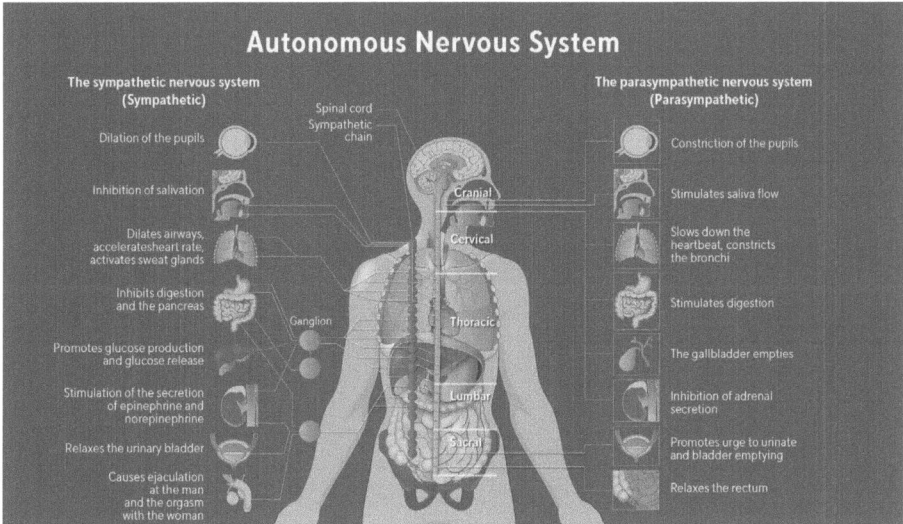

## Vagus Nerve

The vagus nerve is one of twelve cranial nerves and, together with others, originates from the brain stem. It is responsible for controlling the parasympathetic nervous system. The vagus nerve has two main branches - the ventral, which runs through the lungs and heart, and the dorsal, which runs through the back of the lungs and heart as well as all the abdominal organs.

So when we say that singing, facial massages or neck massages are done to relax the vagus nerve, this is not entirely correct. This is because we are stimulating the other cranial nerves. These also have originate in the brain stem. This influences them via the vagus nerve. For example, if we relax the jaw muscles, the tension and pressure in the region is reduced, which can lead to better relaxation of the vagus nerve. This gives the vagus nerve more space to supply the nerve pathways in the forebrain area.

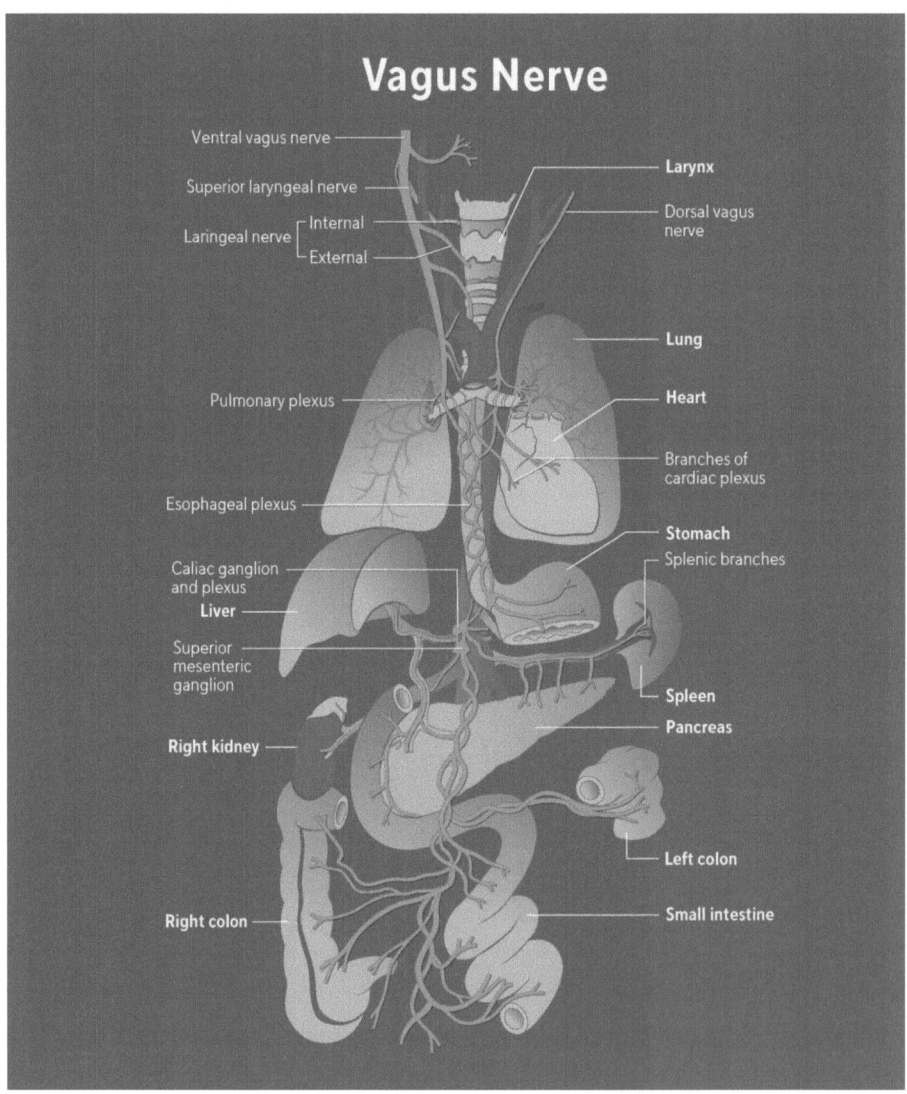

# Emotional Component

Breathing plays a central role in regulating our emotions and can be seen as a mirror of our inner state. Every emotion, be it joy, fear, sadness or anger, has a characteristic influence on our breathing patterns. When we feel stressed or anxious, our breathing tends to become shallower and faster, whereas when we are calm and relaxed, our breathing becomes slower and deeper.

By consciously noticing our breathing, we can recognise what state we are currently in. The quality and pattern of our breathing gives us clues as to whether we are in the ventral vagus area, which is associated with calm and relaxation, the sympathetic area, which is associated with stress and tension, or the dorsal vagus area, which is associated with feelings of sadness, isolation and rigidity.

A simple way to assess our emotional state based on our breathing is to use a scale (see chapter Wave, page 43). By observing our breathing and sensing our body space, we can determine whether we are in a state of calm and serenity or whether we are feeling stressed and anxious.

By noticing our breathing and, if necessary, regulating ourselves through targeted breathing exercises, we can positively influence our mood and reduce unconscious stress.

# Stress Breathing, Overbreathing and Hyperacidity

Overbreathing, known in its extreme form as hyperventilation, occurs when someone breathes deeper and faster than necessary. This can easily happen, especially when trying to take a deep breath or when stressed. This can lead to a disturbance of biochemical balance and acidification of the blood due to a decrease in carbon dioxide levels. Normally our body carefully regulates the pH value of the blood, but this process can be disturbed during overbreathing. Acidification of the blood can cause symptoms such as dizziness, light-headedness, muscle cramps and even unconsciousness.

Interestingly, the body tries to protect you from this type of breathing by making you feel like you're not getting any air, even though you're actually inhaling too much.

An average person breathes in and out about 6 to 9 litres of air per minute, which is enough for an adequate oxygen supply. In contrast, an asthmatic may inhale 15 to 18 litres per minute due to breathing difficulties or stress and still feel like they are not getting enough air.

The solution is to cultivate a gentler, quieter and more natural way of breathing. Through more conscious breathing techniques, such as slow and silent breathing, the body can regain its balance. Relaxation promotes an optimal oxygen supply and also reduces stress and anxiety.

Stress breathing means breathing into the chest, inhaling more than exhaling, often through the mouth. The breath moves in the chest area, we often breathe through the mouth, more in than out.

Stress breathing leads to hyperacidity, which can result in silent inflammation and chronic illnesses.

## The Anatomical Processes of Breathing

The interrelationships and mode of action of the breath are extremely complex. In this book, we start with the anatomical aspects so that we can then go into more detail on the psychosocial level. The more extensive your background knowledge, the more natural the integration of breathing awareness into your everyday life will become.

**Anatomy**

The respiratory centre is a functional unit in the brain located in the medulla oblongata made up of different nerve cells.

The autonomic nervous system sets the pace for breathing. The sympathetic nervous system controls inhalation. It widens the airways and increases the respiratory rate. The parasympathetic nervous system controls exhalation. The airways narrow and the respiratory rate decreases.

**Inhalation is an Active, Sympathicotonic Process.**

During ideal inhalation (abdominal or diaphragmatic breathing), the diaphragm lowers towards the abdomen and the intercostal muscles tense. The lungs passively follow this movement and expand. Now they can fill with fresh air. At the same time, the sinking diaphragm massages the abdominal organs. Breathing helps digestion. The pulse increases with every inhalation.

**Breathing Out is a Passive, Parasympathetic Process.**

The outer intercostal muscles relax. The lungs contract, causing air rich in carbon dioxide to be exhaled. The pulse rate drops with each exhalation.

If stress, a change in posture (due to excessive mobile phone use, hard physical work or illness), emotions, drug use, obesity and neuronal diseases make breathing difficult, breathing changes. This has serious consequences for the whole system.

You can consciously exhale forcefully (forced exhalation). This involves using the abdominal muscles to push the abdominal viscera upwards and thus push the diaphragm upwards.

# External and Internal Breathing

Breathing is the vital process by which oxygen is absorbed from the air (external respiration) and transported to all body cells, where it is used to generate energy (internal respiration). This produces water and carbon dioxide. The latter is released into the exhaled air in the lungs. But how does human respiration work in detail?

**External Respiration**

External respiration (pulmonary respiration) takes place in the lungs. It refers to the intake of oxygen from the air we breathe and the release of carbon dioxide into the air we breathe. The whole process is controlled by the respiratory centre in the brain. In detail, external respiration takes place as follows:

Oxygen-rich air flows through the mouth, nose and throat into the windpipe, where it is warmed, moistened and purified on its way. From the trachea, it continues into the bronchi and their smaller branches, the bronchioles. At the end of the bronchioles, the air we breathe enters the approximately 300 million air sacs (alveoli). These have very thin walls and are surrounded by a network of very fine blood vessels (capillaries). This is where the gas exchange takes place (as follows):

The oxygen in the air we breathe diffuses through the membrane of the alveoli into the blood, where it binds to haemoglobin (red blood pigment in the red blood cells). At the same time, carbon dioxide diffuses from the blood into the alveoli and is then exhaled with the air.

Haemoglobin transports the bound oxygen with the bloodstream to all organs and cells that need it for energy production.

**Internal Respiration**

Internal respiration is also known as **tissue respiration or cellular respiration**. It describes the biochemical process by which organic substances are changed (oxidised) with the help of oxygen in order to release the energy stored in the substances and make it usable in the form of ATP (adenosine triphosphate). ATP is the most important form of energy storage within cells.

Carbon dioxide is produced during internal respiration. It is transported from the blood into the lungs and partially exhaled there (as part of external respiration).

# Lung Capacity

Improving lung capacity is an important part of a healthy lifestyle. Expanding lung capacity and breathing volume through mindful breathing and relaxation can also be supported by medical examinations such as a lung function test. Spirometry is one such test that gives us information about lung capacity and respiratory volume. During the test, you breathe through a mouthpiece into a special device that measures the airflow and the amount of air that flows in and out of the lungs.

To promote lung capacity, it is essential that the following muscles are stretched and strengthened:

**Respiratory Muscles**
These muscles include the diaphragm and the intercostal muscles.

**Accessory Respiratory Muscles**
These muscles include some muscles of the neck and chest muscles and the abdominal muscles. They can support inspiration or expiration.

Testing and improving lung capacity is important for the following reasons:

**Health Benefits**
Good lung capacity is the basis for health and lightness. Improved lung function can reduce the risk of respiratory diseases such as asthma, COPD (chronic obstructive pulmonary disease) and pneumonia.

**Improved Endurance**
Greater lung capacity enables the body to absorb more oxygen and utilise it more efficiently. This improves endurance and physical performance during sporting activities.

**Better Stress Management**
By controlling and deepening your breathing, relaxation techniques such as mindfulness exercises and breathing techniques can help to reduce stress and promote inner calm.

**Improved Quality of Life**
Improved lung capacity helps us to feel less tired and exhausted in everyday life. We are better able to cope with physical exertion without getting out of breath, which improves our overall quality of life.

**Prevention of Illness**
Regular training of the respiratory muscles and improving lung capacity can help to reduce the risk of cardiovascular disease and other chronic illnesses.

The combination of breath focussing and relaxation techniques can help patients to feel calm and relaxed during the test, which can lead to more accurate measurement results. In addition, these techniques can help you to concentrate on the flow of breath and maintain even breathing.

Overall, the combination of conscious breathing, relaxation techniques and medical examinations can help to improve breathing volume and therefore fitness.

The inspiratory, expiratory and residual volume table shows different volumes of lung function that are important measures of respiratory physiology.

Incidentally, the surface area of the alveoli, through which gas exchange takes place, covers a total area of 50 to 100 square metres. That is around fifty times more than the surface area of the body.

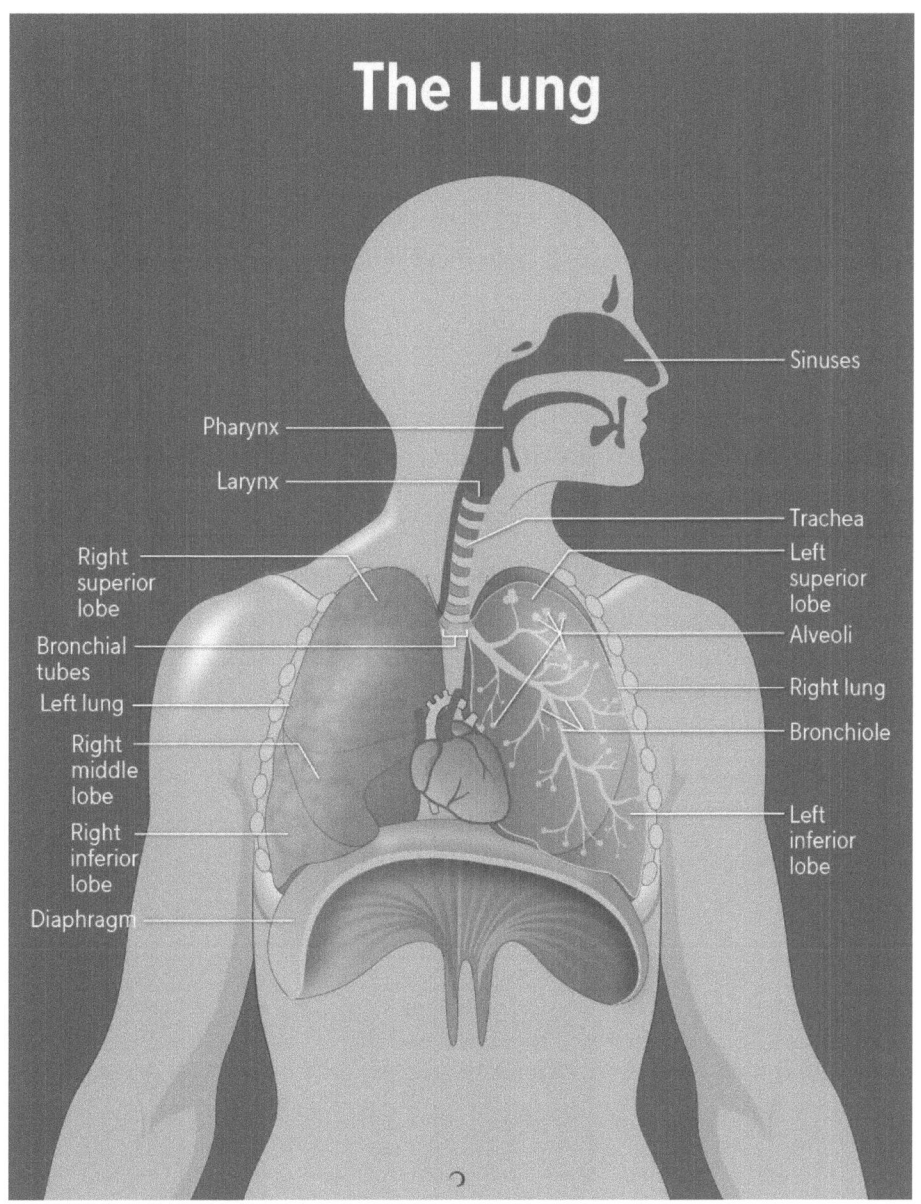

The Lung

Sinuses

Pharynx

Larynx

Trachea

Left superior lobe

Right superior lobe

Alveoli

Bronchial tubes

Left lung

Right lung

Right middle lobe

Bronchiole

Right inferior lobe

Left inferior lobe

Diaphragm

### Inspiratory Volume (IV)

The inspiratory volume is the amount of air that is inhaled during a normal breath without the need for additional effort. This volume varies according to age, gender and physical condition.

### Expiratory Volume (EV)

The expiratory volume is the amount of air that is exhaled after a normal breath without additional effort. It is important for determining lung function and can vary depending on individual factors.

### Residual Volume (RV)

The residual volume is the amount of air that remains in the lungs after maximum exhalation and cannot be exhaled. It serves to protect the lungs from collapsing and is an important component of lung function.

The table may contain different values for these volumes, which may vary depending on individual characteristics and health status. Measuring and analysing these volumes is important for assessing respiratory physiology and can help in the diagnosis and treatment of respiratory diseases and in monitoring lung function.

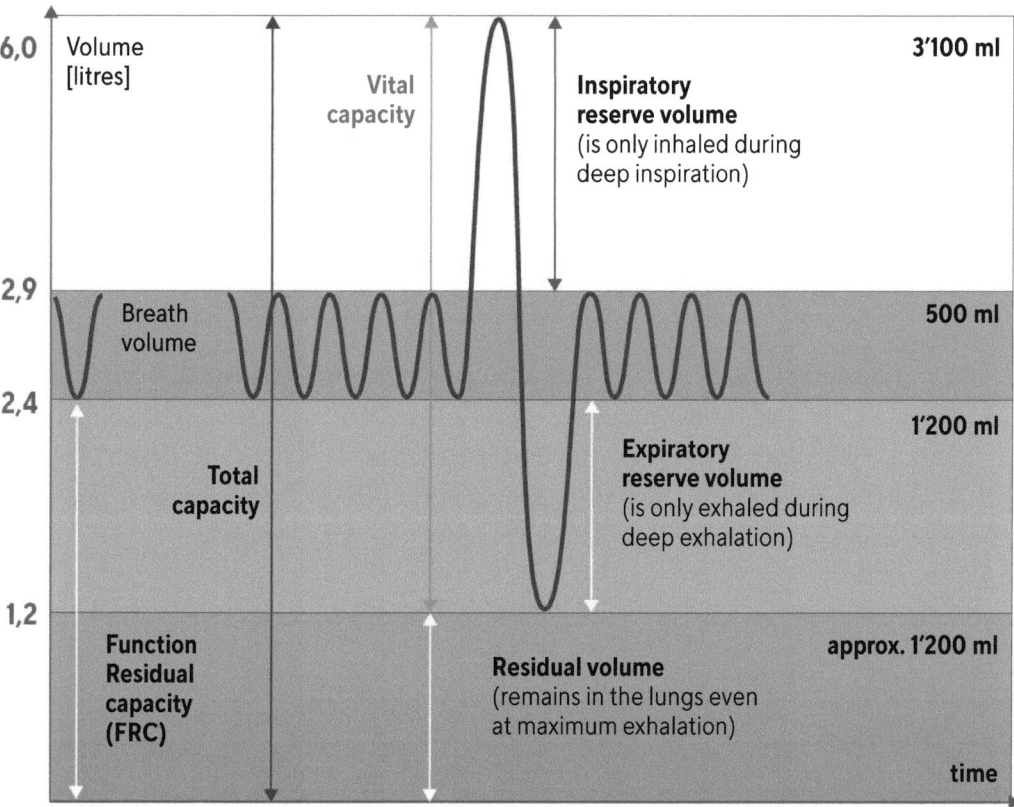

Volume [litres]

6,0 — 3'100 ml

Vital capacity

**Inspiratory reserve volume** (is only inhaled during deep inspiration)

2,9 — 500 ml

Breath volume

2,4 — 1'200 ml

**Total capacity**

**Expiratory reserve volume** (is only exhaled during deep exhalation)

1,2 — approx. 1'200 ml

**Function Residual capacity (FRC)**

**Residual volume** (remains in the lungs even at maximum exhalation)

time

## Polyvagal Theory

The polyvagal theory according to Dr. Stephen Porges explains that our autonomic nervous system has three levels:

**The ventral branch of the vagus nerve stands for safety, connectedness, social integration and interaction (green area).**

**The sympathetic nervous system is responsible for activity, fight and flight (red area).**

**The dorsal branch of the vagus nerve is responsible for collapse, freeze and relaxation (blue area).**

Even during periods of rest, the sympathetic nervous system or dorsal vagus can be chronically activated, which means stress for our ANS and has long-term effects on our health. Numerous studies have shown the connection between stress and life expectancy and disease development. Ideally, the ventral vagus nerve is harmoniously active and responsible for relaxation, digestion, social integration, joy and empathy.

## Wave

When I saw the graphic of this wave, the world became round for me. With this simple illustration, I was finally able to demonstrate breathing therapy and the effects of the breath and explain them to people in an understandable way. It forms the centrepiece, the foundation of my work, which I always work out with all clients first. Self-assessment of one's own, often unconscious, state has top priority.

The three areas shown in different colours in the diagram are explained in more detail below and illustrated with examples.

**VAGUS FLOW°**

# The Wave

Based on Porges' polyvagal theory, I created this wave, which is a valuable working tool:

This graphic illustrates the three areas of vagal tone and its influence on our lives and our physical and mental state. Users learn to assess themselves according to the scale and use appropriate interventions to return to the desired state.

**The behavioral cascade proceeds as follows:**

**8 - 10**  **Life-threatening**
the signals are classified as life-threatening - dorsal vagus branch in the parasympathetic nervous system

**4 - 7**  **Danger**
the signals are classified as danger - sympathetic nervous system

**1 - 3**  **Security**
the signals are classified as safe - ventral vagus in the parasympathetic nervous system

**DORSAL VAGUS IN THE PARASYMPATHETIC**
Darkness, mind wandering, being at the mercy of others, worry, loss of body awareness, dullness, pain, withdrawal, apathy, flaccidity, listlessness, ignorance, negativity, passivity, brooding, senselessness, coldness

**SYMPATHIC TONE**
Withdrawal, restlessness, aggression, activity, attack, loss of physical sensation, addiction, passion, craving for substances, egotism, tunnel vision, sensory change, urge to move, search, increased perception, excitement

**VENTRAL VAGUS IN THE PARASYMPATHETIC**
Pleasure, creativity, intelligence, empathy, relaxation, regeneration, harmony, flow, goodwill, cooperation, peace, access to own abilities and competences, security, friendliness, play, sovereignty, resilience

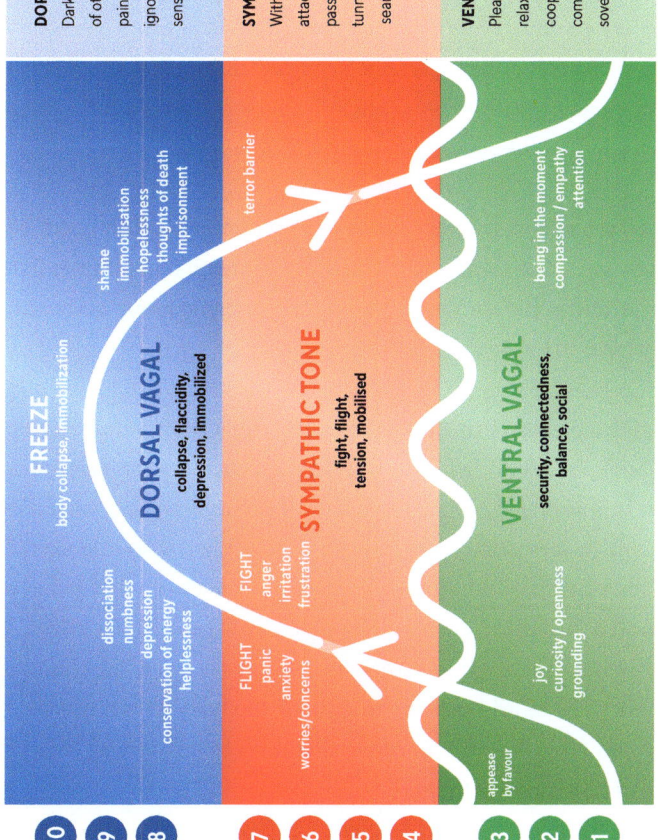

**FREEZE**
body collapse, immobilization

**DORSAL VAGAL**
collapse, flaccidity,
depression, immobilized

shame
immobilisation
hopelessness
thoughts of death
imprisonment

terror barrier

**SYMPATHIC TONE**
fight, flight,
tension, mobilised

**VENTRAL VAGAL**
security, connectedness,
balance, social

being in the moment
compassion / empathy
attention

dissociation
numbness
depression

conservation of energy
helplessness

**FIGHT**
anger
irritation
frustration

**FLIGHT**
panic
anxiety
worries/concerns

joy
curiosity / openness
grounding

appease
by favour

10  9  8

7  6  5  4

3  2  1

VAGUS FLOW© Theory· 2023

## Ventral Vagus – Green Area

We feel completely content, at ease and safe in our environment. The predominant feeling is joy, curiosity and openness. Our brain is relaxed, the limbic system functions perfectly.

We can empathise, sympathise, our face is relaxed, we laugh with our eyes. We regulate ourselves through contact with our fellow human beings. When stress impulses occur, we first seek eye contact. If our fellow human beings remain calm, we immediately regulate ourselves back into relaxation. In this state, we are creative and intuitive, we can draw from the depths. With a pinch of the sympathetic nervous system, we are also active enough to realise our visions, dreams and plans to a healthy degree.

In the green area, we feel what we need, have a great sense of our body and know when we are hungry or tired and need islands of calm. We like being alone, which is a big difference to being lonely. We need this retreat to refuel, rest and recharge our batteries. The breath moves, dynamically, sometimes a little higher, sometimes a little lower, just like the muscles and facial expressions.

The breath adapts to every thought, every emotion. The heart is the first to recognise danger and sends signals to the brain. The breath reacts immediately, much faster than we can think. Before we are aware of the danger, our body has already reacted and adapted to the external situation.

Imagine a person sitting on a park bench on a calm, sunny day, engrossed in the pages of a book. Suddenly, without warning, a sharp, vibrating sensation jolts through their body. It is as if an invisible wave has hit her directly and passed through her. This feeling, which seems to come from deep inside her, is so intense that it makes her heart beat faster a second before her mind even realises what is happening. Then, with a fraction of a delay after this feeling has overwhelmed her senses, the resounding bang reaches her ears. Lightning had struck not far away, the thunder so powerful that it was not only heard but felt throughout the body. It is a moving example of how our body can react to extreme external stimuli by perceiving them before our conscious self can fully process them.

# Sympathetic Nervous System – Red Area

We need a certain amount of activity to realise our projects and actions. This means that we leave the green area and enter the red area a little, but only up to level 5. As this 5th level is still healthy, but already belongs to the sympathetic area, the red area, in contrast to the other 2 areas, has 4 instead of just 3 levels.

If the stress increases further, from level 5 or 6, the entire stress cascade comes into play. (see diagram of the vegetative nervous system on page 31) When we perceive stress or a stress impulse, we first try to regulate ourselves in the green area via our environment. If this is not successful, the stress initially appears harmless - a little concern, worry, frustration or irritation.

If the stress level continues to rise, this means that the fear, panic, anger and rage turn into a flight or fight response.

Tension increases, the liver releases sugar to strengthen the muscles. We lose body awareness because we have no time for pain. The blood thickens so that the wound heals more quickly in the event of an injury. The bronchial tubes are widened so that we can take in more air. Breathing rises up into the chest region and is emphasised, abdominal breathing is reduced. The pupils dilate, we see different things than in the green area and we hear different frequencies with our ears. Our senses are sharpened to the extreme so that we can react more quickly if danger approaches us, such as a dangerous animal (lion) or a violent person.

The following situations from our professional or private lives can also put us in similar situations:

· We have a toxic relationship with a superior or life partner and he again criticises us severely, not only factually but also personally.

· We are travelling alone on what should be a safe mountain tour and are unexpectedly surprised by a storm with snowfall and are afraid that we will not reach our accommodation before nightfall.

· In his absence, the supervisor asks us to explain certain topics to the management board in 20 minutes. However, we are talking for life, let alone in front of the company's highest committee.

· Making an appearance on a big stage.

The limbic system - the emotions - are reduced, including empathy, for example. This was a topic that occupied me for a very long time. We humans have learnt to use empathy as a strategy because we should have compassion. But when we are stressed, we can't really feel it from the depths. It is simply a behaviour that has made us survive. Empathy is reduced because we can't empathise with our opponent in combat. When we see our opponent as a human being or see the animal we are fighting as a sentient being, this blockage of human empathy occurs. The problem with this is often that we have not learnt how to deal with strong emotions appropriately. That's why they become threatening and overwhelming for us. Men are more likely to act loud, angry, furious and aggressive, while women have been trained to be calm, kind and gentle. On the other hand, men should not cry or give up, but should always be strong. The brain reacts immediately when emotional overstimulation occurs. We are catapulted into the blue zone faster than we can think.

Before we get to the blue zone, I would like to mention here that people who have anchored their feet in the green zone can surf up and down this wave. They quickly find their way back into the relaxed zone. It is normal for us to move into the red and blue zones (Read more about this topic on page 60).

Depending on what moves us personally, our state can change.
Here are a few examples:

· I have to write an exam or give a presentation.

· I'm not feeling well, I've had my blood tested and am now awaiting a diagnosis.

· I unexpectedly bump into an unpleasant person.

· I crash my bike, am in pain and in shock.

· The newborn cries a disproportionate amount and I don't know why.

· I'm on a rollercoaster and get scared.

# Dorsal Vagus – Blue Area

The predominant basic feeling is sadness, up to and including depression, whereby in a depression one can also be completely numb and no longer perceive the sadness. This can lead to a freeze reflex. This can be illustrated well using the example of posture. From standing upright and tensing the muscles, you collapse forwards, similar to the mobile phone posture, in which the dorsal vagus nerve puts the muscles at the back of the body into a kind of armadillo reflex to protect yourself from attack.

The energy that was previously used for fighting and mobilisation is now directed against itself. We go into introversion, the breath becomes superficial. The more superficial the breath, the greater the stress. The eyes wander, the head carousel spins incessantly, but the body sensation has practically disappeared, to the point of complete dissociation, where we hardly feel anything. Thoughts circle senselessly, feelings range from shame to thoughts of death and absolute hopelessness. The body is limp, we think, but we cannot mobilise.

This area also has another function, namely deep relaxation, which is experienced without stress and is controlled by the dorsal vagus nerve. For example, when cuddling, when we let ourselves fall into the arms of our partner and feel safe and secure and can immerse ourselves in the deepest relaxation. In the negative state, we feel lonely and isolated, a big difference to the green area, where there is joy and we can happily withdraw and be alone. Here in the blue zone we feel insecure and people cannot offer us sufficient regulation because the social system is threatening. We may shiver, feel cold and see no way out of the situation, at its mercy. The body becomes immobile and we commit self-harming acts.

Many people find themselves trapped in relationships that are not actually good for them, or remain in work relationships or religious communities that offer them supposed security and structure in order to be able to relax better on the outside.

We fall prey to mechanisms that we know are harmful, for example: We consume bad substances, eat junk food in front of the television instead of going for a walk, meeting friends, being creative and enjoying life.

**The biggest challenge of all is this stage,
which I call the terror barriers.**

## Terror Barrier

We awaken from the blue zone. We very much want to return to the state of relaxation. However, we cannot jump over the terror barrier in the red zone (see in the red zone, on the right, on the way back to the green zone). In doing so, we come closer to this zone, sniffing the air, which is peppered with anxiety, panic attacks, feelings of loneliness and abandonment. At first, the physical and psychological symptoms may worsen.

We had already experienced an emotional sensory overload on the way up to the blue zone and it is precisely these feelings that are waiting for us here in the terror barrier. It's as if sabre-toothed tigers were lurking in the bushes everywhere and attacking us. Many of us need professional help and/or a very understanding environment to guide us through this death zone.

If this is not the case, we sniff the air and immediately return to the blue zone because it is more pleasant, less emotional and supposedly safer.

We stay there until we make the next attempt and fail again at the terror barrier. The good news, however, is that we develop more confidence in ourselves every time we cross this terror barrier. Namely, the confidence that we can manage every single panic attack, which supposedly means death, is manageable. It gradually becomes a little better, safer and more trusting. Orientation becomes more focussed and we are on the direct path home, on the way, into the green zone.

**Summary**

In the VAGUS FLOW® method, we focus on being in the now and mindfully observing what is happening. This practice strengthens our awareness of our own breath and body awareness, which helps us to recognise unhealthy behavioural patterns and distance ourselves from them. VAGUS FLOW® is a simple but powerful method for recognising unconscious emotions and reducing stress.

Through conscious breathing, we activate the ventral vagus nerve, which relaxes us and helps to alleviate symptoms of various stress states. The aim is to put us in a state where we feel safe and healthy and are open to social interaction. It is essential to strengthen our resilience so that we can face life's challenges more calmly.

People often fail due to a lack of healthy social connections, injuries and traumas. Just like healing, they do not happen in isolation.

From this chapter, we can see how crucial healthy social connections are to our healing. By learning to maximise social safety, joy and curiosity in our lives, we find a place of inner strength and peace - our own bodies. A robust nervous system allows us to deal with stress without falling into patterns of avoidance or withdrawal.

This teaching helps us to learn practical tools and techniques that we can integrate into our daily lives to respond more consciously and calmly to stressors. These everyday applications not only help us to remain calm in moments of tension, but also promote a deeper and lasting change in the way we deal with challenges and interpersonal relationships.

# Stress

This chapter is about how our body reacts to stress and why it is important to learn and apply stress management techniques. A better understanding of the role of adrenaline, noradrenaline and cortisol can help us to deal with stress more consciously and protect our health in the long term.
*See illustration Autonomous Nervous System, page 31*

Prolonged stress not only puts a strain on our psyche, but also has a negative effect on our body. In times of stress, our body switches to alert mode. Heart rate, breathing and blood pressure increase, blood sugar levels rise, the bronchial tubes dilate and our immune system is briefly activated. This mechanism is very useful in acute situations in order to cope with challenges. However, if stress becomes a permanent condition, it can cause serious health problems.

## Chronic Stress and its Consequences
Chronic stress can lead to a variety of serious illnesses, including cardiovascular disease, gastrointestinal problems, diabetes, burn-out syndrome and mental disorders such as depression and many more.

The way we breathe plays an important role in this. In stressful situations, many people tend to breathe shallowly and quickly, which can increase the body's alertness. Through natural breathing, however, we can activate the parasympathetic part of our nervous system, which is responsible for relaxation and recovery. This helps us to reduce stress and the negative effects of chronic stress on our body and mind.

The body goes through **three phases** of the stress response:

In the **alarm reaction phase,** more stress hormones are released to prepare the body for the challenge.

In the **resistance phase**, the body tries to adapt to the prolonged stress situation, which often leads to typical stress symptoms such as high blood pressure or tension.

Finally, the **exhaustion phase** leads to a feeling of being overwhelmed, a decrease in performance and an increased risk of illnesses such as colds or mental disorders.

The first physical and psychological signs of stress are manifold: tension, headaches, stomach problems, sleep problems, concentration problems and mood swings are just some of them.

„Stress makes you addicted
to even more stress".

**Brain Reactions to Stress**

When the stress cascade is triggered in the brain, a complex series of reactions occur that affect several areas of the brain, including the limbic system. The limbic system is responsible for processing emotions, memories and the survival of relevant information.

„Learn to relax and you will hear
the sound of your innermost dreams again."

# Stress System

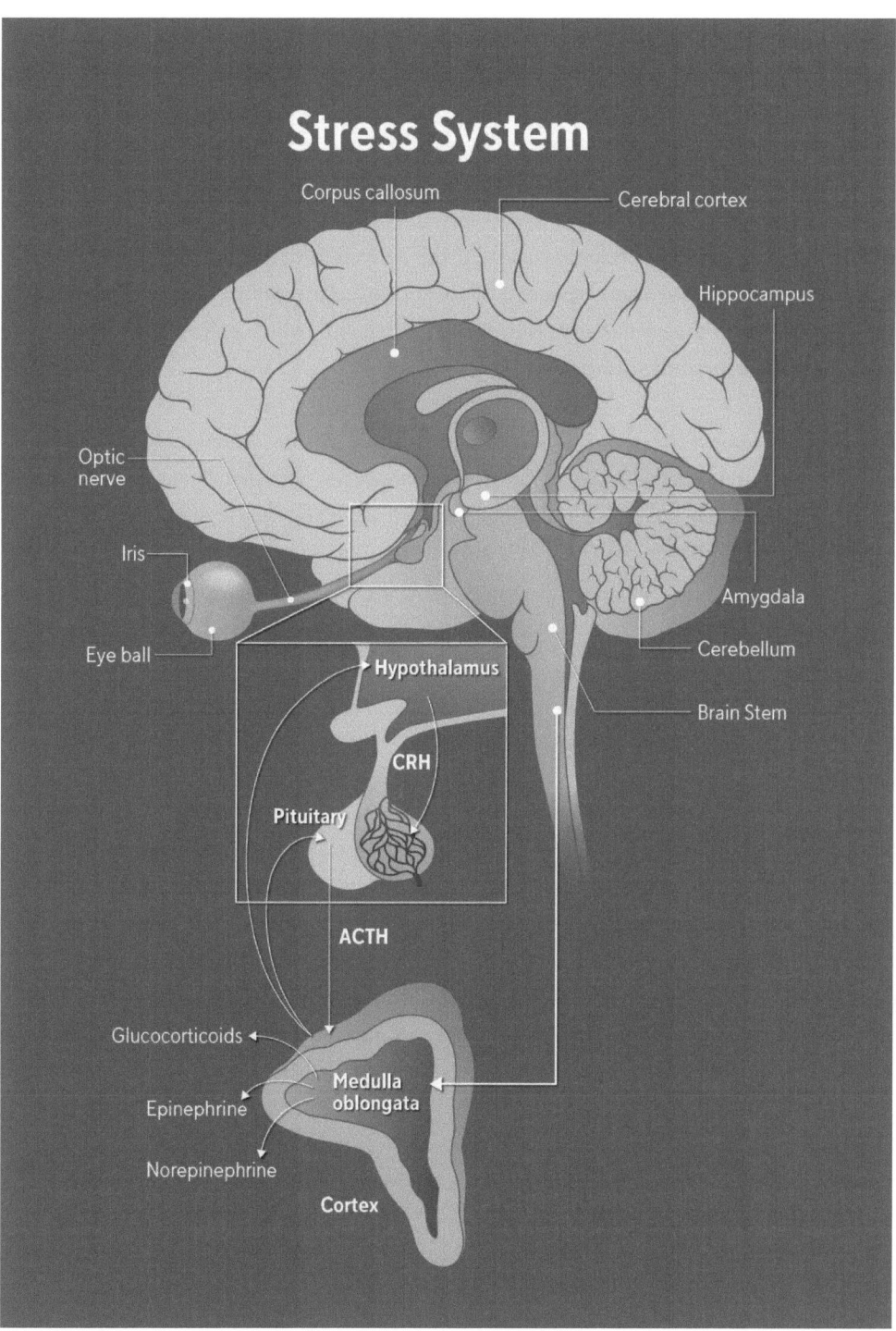

Corpus callosum

Cerebral cortex

Hippocampus

Optic nerve

Iris

Eye ball

Amygdala

Cerebellum

Brain Stem

Hypothalamus

CRH

Pituitary

ACTH

Glucocorticoids

Epinephrine

Medulla oblongata

Norepinephrine

Cortex

# „Avoid following stress-driven impulses that confuse the melody of dreams with illusion."

The first step in the stress response is often the activation of the amygdala, a core structure in the limbic system. The amygdala acts as an „alarm centre" and recognises potential threats. It then sends signals to the hypothalamus, which plays a key role in controlling the autonomic nervous system.

The hypothalamus activates the sympathetic branch of the autonomic nervous system, which prepares the body for the stress response. At the same time, the hypothalamus releases corticotropin-releasing hormone (CRH), which stimulates the release of adrenocorticotropin (ACTH) from the pituitary gland.

ACTH reaches the adrenal cortex and stimulates the release of cortisol, an important stress hormone.

Adrenaline is also released by the sympathetic nervous system and the adrenal medulla.

During these processes, various parts of the limbic system, such as the amygdala and the hippocampus, are activated. The hippocampus plays a role in the regulation of stress reactions and the processing of memory content. It produces these neurones in a relaxed, joyful state - until the end of our lives. This enables us to create fresh neuronal highways, learn new behavioural patterns and courageously tread unknown paths. While the amygdala evaluates the emotional significance of events and influences the body's reaction to them.

**In Summary**, activation of the stress cascade leads to a complex neuroendocrine and physiological response mediated by the interaction of multiple brain regions, including the limbic system.

*These hormones and their sites of production are critical to the regulation of numerous bodily functions, from stress response to metabolism, growth and reproduction.*

## Hormones

When we are under stress, our body activates the sympathetic state, a response that prepares us for challenges. This state is controlled by the sympathetic nervous system, which works like an emergency switch to put us on alert. Two hormones in particular come into play here: adrenaline and noradrenaline.

Adrenaline increases your heart rate, expands your lungs to take in more oxygen and ensures that more blood flows to your muscles. It literally makes you ready for a quick reaction - be it flight or confrontation. Noradrenaline supports adrenaline, mainly by increasing your blood pressure to ensure that all parts of your body are well supplied. Another important player in this scenario is cortisol. This hormone helps to release energy by breaking down fats and sugars, ensuring you have enough energy to respond to prolonged stress. In the short term, cortisol can actually be useful as it has an anti-inflammatory effect and supports the immune system. If this state lasts too long and cortisol is constantly released in high amounts, it can lead to negative effects such as a weakened immune system, increased blood pressure and other stress-related health problems. It also inhibits the hippocampus, meaning it affects the production of happy neurons.

## Hormone Production

Hormones are produced in various organs and tissues throughout the body. Here is a brief overview of some of the most important hormones and where they are produced (see diagram).

**Adrenaline and Noradrenaline** are produced in the adrenal glands, more specifically in the adrenal medulla. These hormones play a central role in the body's response to stress.

**Cortisol,** another stress hormone, is also produced in the adrenal glands, but in the adrenal cortex.

**Insulin and Glucagon**, hormones that regulate blood sugar levels, are produced in the pancreas. Insulin is produced by the beta cells and glucagon by the alpha cells of the islets of Langerhans.

**Thyroxine (T4) and Triiodothyronine (T3),** hormones that influence metabolism, are produced in the thyroid gland.

**Parathyroid Hormone,** which regulates the calcium level in the blood, is produced in the parathyroid glands.

**Testosteron,** the primary male sex hormone, is mainly produced in the testicles in men - in women, a smaller amount is produced in the ovaries and adrenal glands.

**Oestrogen and Progesterone,** the primary female sex hormones, are mainly produced in the ovaries and play an important role in the menstrual cycle and pregnancy. Men also produce a small amount of these hormones, primarily in fatty tissue and the testicles.

**Growth Hormone,** which promotes growth and cell reproduction, is produced in the pituitary gland.

# Endocrine System

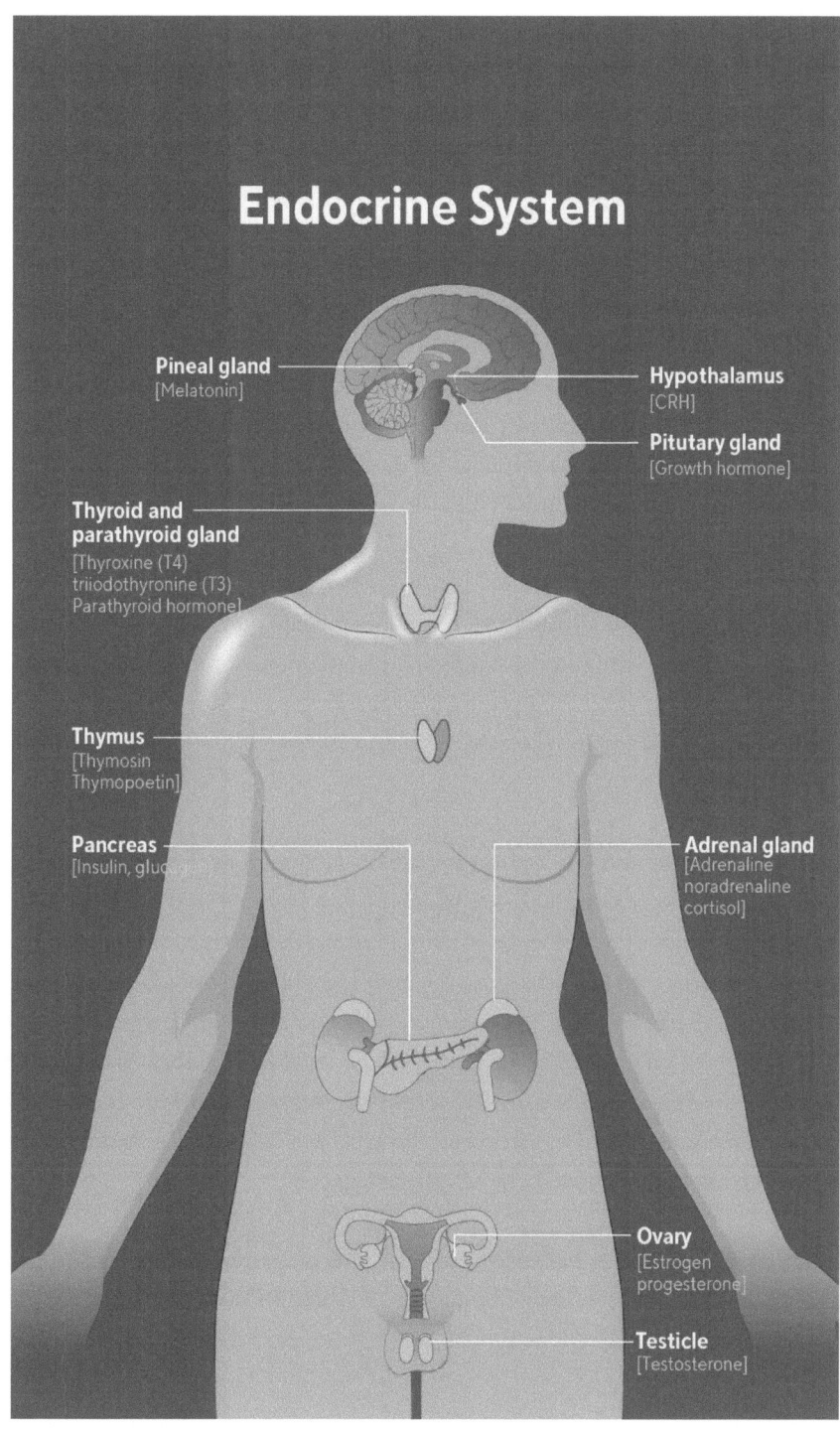

Pineal gland
[Melatonin]

Hypothalamus
[CRH]

Pitutary gland
[Growth hormone]

Thyroid and
parathyroid gland
[Thyroxine (T4)
triiodothyronine (T3)
Parathyroid hormone]

Thymus
[Thymosin
Thymopoetin]

Pancreas
[Insulin, glucagon]

Adrenal gland
[Adrenaline
noradrenaline
cortisol]

Ovary
[Estrogen
progesterone]

Testicle
[Testosterone]

**Chronic Stress and its Influence on Hormone Balance**

Chronic stress is a persistent challenge for the human body and has far-reaching effects on hormonal balance. The constant overproduction of stress hormones such as adrenaline, noradrenaline and, in particular, cortisol, can disrupt the finely tuned balance of our endocrine system. This chapter sheds light on what happens to the hormones during chronic stress and what imbalances and diseases can arise as a result.

**Cortisol and its Long-Term Effects:** Cortisol plays a central role in the response to stress. It helps in the short term by mobilising energy and modulating the immune system. In the case of chronic stress, however, cortisol levels remain high, which can lead to various health problems. A permanently elevated cortisol level can weaken the immune system, disrupt the blood sugar balance and lead to weight gain, especially in the abdominal area. It also increases the risk of cardiovascular disease, type 2 diabetes and can lead to burnout.

**Adrenaline and Noradrenaline:** These hormones prepare the body for rapid reactions. In the case of chronic stress, a constantly increased production leads to a continuous increase in heart rate and blood pressure. In the long term, this can put a strain on the cardiovascular system and increase the risk of hypertension (high blood pressure) and heart disease.

**Progesterone:** Stress also has a direct impact on progesterone, a hormone produced in women, particularly in the ovaries, which plays a key role in the menstrual cycle and pregnancy. Under the influence of chronic stress, the production of progesterone can be impaired. In stressful situations, the body prioritises the production of cortisol in the adrenal glands by using the common precursor hormone, pregnenolone. This phenomenon is often referred to as „pregnenolone stealing" or „cortisol escape". As a result of this diversion, progesterone levels drop. Low progesterone levels can lead to a number of problems, including irregular menstrual cycles, difficulty getting pregnant and, in some cases, an increased risk of miscarriage.

In addition, an imbalance between oestrogen and progesterone can lead to conditions such as PMS (premenstrual syndrome) and PMDD (premenstrual dysphoric disorder).

In view of these correlations, it becomes clear how important effective stress management is for maintaining a healthy hormonal balance and, in particular, for the health of the female reproductive system.

**Effects on other Hormone Systems:** The permanent activation of the sympathic nervous system and the high concentration of stress hormones can also affect the production and function of other hormones. For example, an imbalance in the production of thyroid hormones can occur, leading to metabolic disorders. Reproductive hormones such as testosterone, oestrogen and progesterone can also be affected, which can impair fertility and lead to cycle disorders.

**Mental Health:** In addition to the physical effects, chronic stress also has a significant impact on mental health. It can increase the risk of anxiety disorders and depression, which in turn can exacerbate dysfunctional hormone regulation.

**Coping Strategies:** To minimise the negative effects of chronic stress on hormone balance and health, it is crucial to develop effective stress management strategies. These include regular breath observation and mindfulness practice, such as physical activity, adequate sleep, a balanced diet and building a supportive social network. The best way to regulate stress is to promote and cultivate joy.

To summarise, this chapter shows how chronic stress can disrupt hormonal balance and lead to a variety of health problems. By learning to regulate your stress and adjust your lifestyle accordingly, you will have a positive effect on the whole organism. Stress, especially unconscious stress, is the foundation for chronic illness on both a physical and psychological level.

## Natural Stress Curve

There is a fascinating example in the animal world that can teach us a lot about how to deal with stress. Imagine a herd of flight animals, such as antelopes, grazing peacefully. These animals are constantly alert and keep raising their heads to monitor their surroundings. This heightened alertness allows them to relax and enjoy the peace and quiet. This state is often referred to as „rest and digest", as the animals feel safe as long as they are in the group.

However, when danger threatens, these flight animals run away in a flash, as the name suggests. They will not try to fight a lion, but flee. The entire organism releases stress hormones to make the animals as fast, reactive and agile as possible. The lion has usually already selected the weakest animal in the herd and attacks it. This animal has no chance of fighting or fleeing further, so it drops down. This reflex to play dead is one of the oldest reflexes from the brain stem.

Our system is ingeniously organised because the lion is not a scavenger. This means that the animal that drops has a real chance of survival, as the lion is no longer interested in it. It gets up and shakes itself. This shaking is important for survival, because all the stress that was previously produced is released from the body. The animal returns to its family, eats, rests and regains its strength. This is the natural stress curve.

Research has shown that if an animal does not shake itself after an attack or stress, the chance of survival decreases significantly because the stress remains in the body and the immune system is attacked. As a result, the animal either falls ill or, because the predator recognises the weakening immediately, it is attacked and eaten again the next moment.

The problem in our society is that with a chronic stress curve, this release by shaking or trembling does not happen. The stress remains in the body. We also do too little to promote the state of „rest and digest". This results in persistent stress patterns that promote hyperacidity and prepare the ground for silent inflammation and chronic illnesses.

# „He is not brave who knows no fear; he is brave who knows fear and overcomes it."

Khalil Gibran

## Fear

Fear is a natural and normal reaction of the body to potential threats or dangers. It serves as a protective mechanism to ensure your survival in the worst-case scenario. However, when feelings of anxiety become overwhelming and persistent, they can become a burden and severely interfere with daily life.

Anxiety can come in many forms, from mild discomfort to intense panic attacks. It can be caused by various triggers such as stress, triggers, traumatic events, genetic pre-disposition or neurochemical imbalances. The symptoms of anxiety can be physical, such as palpitations, sweating, trembling and stomach discomfort, or psychological, such as worry, fear and negative thoughts.

Anxiety is often a subtle emotion that can manifest itself in different ways. One interesting aspect is that people are not even aware that they are experiencing anxiety, as the brain quickly switches to „fight or flight" mode without conscious thought. This automatic reaction of the brain can lead to feelings of anxiety being suppressed or overlooked as the focus is on coping with the perceived threat. Many people in my practice are convinced that they do not experience anxiety. For me, this is often an alarm sign, as it indicates a permanent and unconscious slide into activity (red area) or freeze (blue area). If you look at the graph of the wave, you can see that the body feeling already decreases from about the 5th level and we adopt a completely different behaviour than when we are between levels 1-4.

It is important to recognise that anxiety is not always obvious and can manifest itself in different ways. Some people experience physical symptoms such as palpitations, sweating or trembling, while others feel anxious, nervous or worried without knowing exactly why. These subtle signs of anxiety can be overlooked, resulting in many people not seeking the help they need to deal with their feelings of anxiety.

Often the breath is the only reliable indicator that you are in a state of anxiety. The breath is in the upper range. The breath stops or your breath is taken away and you can't breathe.

By becoming aware of your own emotional states, you can better understand what is going on and take appropriate steps to recognise anxiety. This can make the difference between a life dominated and controlled by fear and a life characterised by courage, serenity and inner strength.

It is important to understand that fear is a normal and natural human emotion that all of us experience. It only becomes a problem when it becomes excessive and interferes with our daily lives. Fortunately, there are various treatments for anxiety, including psychotherapy, physical therapy, natural remedies and relaxation techniques.

The problem in our society is that with a chronic stress curve, this release by shaking or shivering does not happen. The stress remains in the body. We also do too little to promote the state of „rest and digest". Unconscious chronic stress is responsible for many secondary symptoms.

# „Fear knocked, trust opened –
# no one was outside."
Chinese proverb

## Panic Attacks

During the COVID pandemic, I observed in my practice that many people wearing masks were breathing mainly through their mouths and their breathing was superficial. At the same time, the stories of fear and panic increased significantly, and I noticed certain breathing patterns that have persisted to this day. As soon as breathing switches to mouth breathing and overbreathing occurs, feelings of anxiety and panic can be triggered.

Panic attacks are sudden and intense moments of anxiety that can often occur without any recognisable trigger. Our system is thrown out of balance, releasing a flood of stress hormones such as adrenaline. These hormones trigger a „fight or flight" response that puts the body in a state of alert.

The person experiences a variety of physical and emotional symptoms that affect the autonomic nervous system and the brain.

The brain also plays a central role in the development and progression of panic attacks. In situations that are perceived as threatening or dangerous, the brain reacts by activating the limbic system, which is responsible for processing emotions. This activation can lead to a heightened state of alert, which contributes to the symptoms of a panic attack being intensified.

Symptoms such as palpitations, rapid breathing, dizziness, trembling, sweating, chest pain, nausea and the feeling of losing control or going crazy can occur. These symptoms can be extremely frightening and cause the person to isolate themselves or avoid going to certain situations or places for fear of experiencing another panic attack.

Panic attacks are not a sign of weakness, but a natural reaction of the body to stress and anxiety.

With the right support, people who suffer from panic attacks can learn to manage their symptoms, get out of the attacks more quickly and lead a life of safety and protection.

**Recommendation**
During a panic attack, the lungs and bronchial tubes expand and you breathe in more than you breathe out, even though you feel like you can't breathe.
If you are in the middle of an attack, I recommend that you monitor your breathing and do not breathe more deeply, as this can make the attack worse. On the contrary, breathing should be reduced, slowed down and not increased. You can exhale through your pursed lips and inhale through your nose.

At such moments, it is important to get out as quickly as possible. To regain control of your body and your thoughts, immediately do something completely different and distract yourself. This does not mean repressing something; the issue can be dealt with later in a „sober" way. You can then look at your development processes and solve your problems again when you are back in the green zone, in relaxation. The most important thing is to move into a healthy, conducive state in which the brain can react appropriately and you are not driven by stress impulses.

It can be helpful to stand up, wash your hands and face with cold water or even take a cold shower. Drinking tea can have a calming effect. If a sympathetic person is around, talking can help. Kneading hands, patting the body, shaking or dancing. I also recommend reading comics or watching funny films to get out of the state of danger. It is a so-called paradoxical intervention, where you do the opposite of what you would naturally want to do, namely flee or fight.

„We have a limited number of breaths available for this life. How mindfully we use it determines our lifespan."

Chinese tradition

# Trauma

Trauma is a complex and profound experience that can affect a person's emotional, psychological and often physical well-being. In this chapter, we will look in detail at the two basic forms of trauma: Developmental and shock trauma. Both types have different origins and effects on the lives of those affected, but require a deep understanding and a differentiated approach to treatment.

In the following sections, we will take a closer look at the specific characteristics of the two types of trauma. VAGUS FLOW® is a way of helping those affected to recognise the effects and behavioural patterns in everyday life and to find a way of dealing with them. The aim is to reduce unconscious stress and enable a return to the green zone.

### The Developmental Trauma

Every person, and therefore society as a whole, essentially suffers, often unconsciously, from attachment, relationship or developmental trauma - summarised as developmental trauma.

Similar to shock, mechanisms are at work here, but the cause is not a one-off catastrophic experience, but a persistent relationship pattern that parents or carers have towards the child. This happens when the parents are less able to relate and have a lasting destructive effect on the child due to their own traumatisation. It ranges from subtle emotional abuse to raw physical violence.

A child's survival depends entirely on the affection of the parents. All needs, anger, despair or sadness that parents have repressed in themselves are automatically repressed in their child in order to keep them out of their own consciousness.

In essence, it is about two movements of the child - towards separation, autonomy, independence - or towards closeness, connection, needs. The core emotions of anger and sadness are closely linked. We develop survival strategies to deal with the effects of our childhood.

Developmental trauma, attachment trauma or parenting trauma often occur early in life when children are repeatedly exposed to negative experiences that affect their emotional and psychological development. In many families and societies, we learn to control our emotions and suppress our needs in order to function and persevere. These adaptive strategies are often developed out of a need to survive in an environment that does not support or tolerate emotional expression. This can create deep-seated emotional wounds that affect an individual's long-term well-being and interfere with the ability to self-regulate and maintain healthy interpersonal relationships.

Although as adults we are no longer dependent on our parents, we continue to live in these patterns because we are often unaware of them. Awareness of this enables us to step out of these strategies and opens the doors to deep transformation.


**The Shock Trauma**

After a singular, severe, shock-like experience, the body automatically switches to a state of maximum defence readiness, regardless of whether we want it to or not. This natural process mobilises all available energy for extreme physical stress (fight or flight), which makes sense in order to survive in life-threatening situations.

Trauma refers to an exceptional psychological situation triggered by overwhelming events that pose a threat to the life or physical integrity of the person affected or their loved ones. The autonomic nervous system reacts at lightning speed and prepares the body for extreme, rapid action.

Shock trauma occurs when the organism can no longer find its way out of the highly activated state, even though the danger has long since passed.

„Being deeply ashamed of our natural needs or even our entire existence leads to us no longer showing or sharing them with other people, even later as adults. This is the root cause of all relationship problems and therefore the cause of all suffering."

Gopal Norbert Klein

### The Cause of all Suffering

Due to these unconscious mechanisms, a great deal of stress is stored in the ANS. If this stress is not released, a malfunction occurs that produces an overreaction to relatively small stressors.

Post-traumatic stress disorder can develop immediately after a stressful event, but sometimes years later. Typical symptoms include re-experiencing, vegetative over-excitability, avoidance behaviour and negative changes in thoughts and feelings.

Resolution and healing occur when you can relax your ANS and your body and apply this safety and relaxation to social interaction and communication. Sharing your feelings and needs is fundamental and the foundation for healing.

# „Stress hormones sharpen the senses for the material world and encourage addictive behaviour.“

## Addiction

Addiction does not only mean dependence on substances, but also addiction to material goods or to structures that supposedly provide security. Addiction is often well hidden and occurs in many almost invisible areas, such as binge eating, addiction to work, sport or activity. This constantly stimulates our sympathetic nervous system because the feeling of being active, agile and extroverted is simply great - we perform until we drop. Feelings of emptiness, boredom, sadness and restlessness are difficult to bear, and we like to overlay this with our addictive behaviour.

This can work well for a while, until we feel trapped in a hamster wheel where we always have to do something to activate the sympathetic nervous system when we feel empty or exhausted. This is very exhausting and draining.

### The Subtle Addiction to Drama and How it Affects Our Autonomic Nervous System

This book makes it clear that addiction is not limited to the consumption of substances, but manifests itself subtly in various areas of life. A closer look at the graph of the wave makes it clear that addiction influences many aspects of our lives.

As stress levels increase, so does the risk of addiction. This can manifest itself on a physical level through eating disorders, excessive physical activity and excessive shopping. On an emotional level, the danger becomes apparent when people lose themselves in structures such as religions, philosophies or meditation in search of supposed security. Dependence on the opinions of others or authorities such as gurus and therapists also plays a role.

# „The greater the stress, the greater the risk that we will develop addictive behaviour.“

Particularly recognised in our society is the addiction to work, which keeps us trapped in an endless hamster wheel until we fall off the wheel from exhaustion and stay there. Endless scrolling and lingering in virtual worlds puts us in a state of passive consumption that alienates us from reality. Our attention is fragmented, our interpersonal relationships are leaking, while we are drawn deeper and deeper into the maelstrom of the digital world and allow ourselves to be bombarded by external dramas.

Social media is another multifaceted phenomenon that characterises our modern society. Constantly using our smartphones causes our bodies to lean forwards, our foreheads to furrow and our breathing to become shallow. This posture stimulates our state in the dorsal vagal mode and reinforces our addiction.

All forms of addiction feed our stress behaviour and keep us trapped in our internal prison. I call this summarised: **„The addiction to drama.“**

We are often unconsciously in search of drama. Be it in our personal lives, in the media or in interpersonal relationships - the need for exciting events and emotions is omnipresent. But what is actually behind this subtle addiction to drama and what impact does it have on our ANS and hormones?

The pursuit of drama can become a spiral that puts a strain on our ANS. Our body reacts to stressful situations by activating the sympathetic nervous system, which leads to an increase in stress hormones such as cortisol. In the long term, this state of constant arousal can lead to dysregulation of the ANS, which in turn can cause various physical and psychological complaints.

Addictive behaviour influences our hormone balance. In particular, the reward system in our brain, which releases dopamine as a neurotransmitter, plays an important role. Drama and exciting events release dopamine and create a short-term feeling of satisfaction and pleasure. However, excessive consumption of drama can lead to a blunting of this reward system, which can lead to a vicious cycle.

To counteract this subtle addiction to drama and maintain the health of our ANS and endocrine system, it is important to realise how drama affects our lives. Through the VAGUS FLOW® method and other applications that include mindfulness, stress management techniques and the promotion of a balanced lifestyle, we can learn to break free from this addiction and find a healthy balance.

By understanding these mechanisms and actively addressing them, we can support our autonomic nervous system and hormonal balance.

## Exercise

**Recognise your Subtle Addictive Behaviour**
Take plenty of time for this exercise and start to observe yourself very critically in your everyday life. Pay attention to the emotional moments that tempt you to look at your mobile phone, smoke a cigarette, eat sugar, make a phone call or book your next training session or therapy session. Start to differentiate whether you really need this action now for your life, for your development, or whether you are only choosing it to get out of an inner emptiness or need.

Extend these moments of awareness and be longer and longer with your emotions without wanting to change them. Combine this exercise with the breathing exercises in Part 2.

I wish you the courage you need to embark on your inner journey and be in contact with your emotions.
**Emotion also means „to be in motion" - to be alive.**

# Interventions

In the following chapter, as well as in Part 2 of this book, we explore a variety of methods and interventions that can help you find your inner balance and strengthen your resilience. There are numerous approaches that you can try out until you find what suits you 100% - in the moment and for your individual needs. Observing your natural breath provides a solid basis for promoting self-awareness.

By developing your breath awareness and body awareness, you will be able to choose the interventions that best suit your personal well-being and goals. Breathing practice is mainly about experience.

In addition, strong, rhythmic breathing trainings such as Wim Hof, Holotropic practice and Breathwork are valuable methods that you can also use. However, it is important to be aware of the contraindications and to be mindful when using these techniques. When used correctly, they can be effective tools against stress and panic. Make sure that if you practise this in a group, you feel safe and secure.

The breath is always a mirror for the emotional state you are in at that moment. If you learn to observe the breath, you can assess yourself well on the scale of the wave. You can rely 100% on your breath, all other behaviour patterns can be based on deception.

- Is your breath more in the abdomen? This indicates the green area.
- Is your breath more in the chest area, tending towards mouth breathing, emphasised inhalation? This indicates activation of the sympathetic nervous system, the stress mode.
- Is your breath superficial in the throat, or barely noticeable? This indicates the blue area, the freeze mode.

Learn to assess yourself and learn about the intervention options that will help you get back into the green zone.
You can't promote and nurture the green zone enough.

In the world of performance and stress, anxiety, anger, insomnia and restlessness are often the first symptoms. Use your breath and communicate with your nervous system.

Calming your body and mind increases the activation of the ventral vagus nerve. This can create a feeling of safety and security.

Of course, it always takes the whole package and often requires a combination of approaches - psychotherapy, conventional medicine, breathing therapy, naturopathy and more.

## Analysis of the Autonomic Nervous System

The ANS analysis is a measurement that measures various important data about your heart and nervous system. It shows how your heartbeat changes and how active your autonomic nervous system is.
This makes it possible to visualise how the breathing exercises and other treatments (massage, yoga exercises, conversations) affect the ANS.
Other influences, such as alcohol consumption, computer, sleep behaviour, can be measured and the direct effects of this behaviour can be visually explained.

## Various breathing techniques

### Buteyko
The Buteyko method is a breathing technique that aims to optimise breathing by focusing on reducing and controlling the volume of breath. By training with the Buteyko method, people learn to breathe more shallowly and calmly, which can help to increase $CO_2$ levels in the body and improve oxygen transport. This method is often used for treatment of respiratory conditions such as asthma and stress management. It emphasises the importance of calm and efficient breathing.

**Wim Hof**

The Wim Hof method is a breathing technique based on a combination of breath control, cold exposure and mental focussing. By training with the Wim Hof method, people learn to breathe deeply and hold their breath to strengthen their body and improve their immune response. This method is often used to increase energy, reduce stress and promote health. It emphasises the ability of the mind to control the body.

**Holotropic Practice and Breathwork**

These are techniques that focus on the power of breathing to promote consciousness expansion and emotional healing. Through intensive and conscious breathing, levels of consciousness are reached that enable people to flush deeply rooted emotions, traumas and blockages to the surface and release them. These methods are often used for self-exploration, spiritual development and holistic healing. They emphasise the connection between breathing, consciousness and inner growth and offer access to hidden aspects of the self.

# Music, Breath and Movement

The previous chapters have highlighted the essential importance of the vagus nerve and the diverse effects of breath and movement on its regulation. Music, singing and dancing can be used as key components.

**The Powerful Symbiosis of Music**

Music is an artistic force that can be both invigorating and calming, depending on tempo, rhythm and melody. While calm, harmonious sounds activate the parasympathetic branch of the vagus nerve and have a calming While the vagus nerve can unfold its full effect, fast-paced, powerful rhythms are able to address the sympathetic branch and release energy. By skilfully combining both aspects of music, we achieve a holistic harmonisation of the vagus nerve.

### The Union of Breath and Movement

The unity of conscious breathing and physical movement is also important for the regulation of the vagus nerve. By breathing rhythmically, we can stimulate the parasympathetic branch of the nerve and induce a relaxation response. At the same time, physical exercise activates the organism and reduces stress by releasing endorphins and promoting blood circulation.

### Therapeutic Application

In therapeutic practice, we can use this integrative methodology to support people in their various states of regulation. For those who remain exhausted, collapsed and in a freeze state, we first offer relaxing music and gentle breathing to help the body calm down. As soon as the mind and body are ready, we move on to gradually activating the music and movement to release energy and restore vitality.

### The Effect of Singing and Humming on our Nervous System

Another fascinating way to influence the vagus nerve is through singing and humming. These melodic practices have a direct effect on our nervous system. The effect depends on performance and intention.

Singing activates different areas of the brain, including those associated with emotions, memory and reward. This can lead to the release of endorphins, which increase feelings of well-being and happiness. Singing also stabilises the breathing rhythm and harmonises the heart rate.

Similar to singing, humming has a calming effect on the nervous system. The vibrations in the body help to centre the mind and direct thoughts.

### Conclusion

The comprehensive regulation of the vagus nerve through music, breathing and movement requires a balanced interplay of activating and relaxing elements. By taking both aspects into account and integrating them into therapeutic approaches, we promote balance.

Singing and humming are powerful tools. By using them consciously in therapeutic contexts and in everyday life, we can brighten our moods considerably.

# Contraindications

### Cardiovascular Diseases
Dynamic breathing exercises can increase the heart rate and affect blood pressure.

### Respiratory Diseases
People with certain respiratory diseases such as asthma or COPD should be careful, as dynamic breathing exercises can lead to breathlessness or other complications.

### Pregnancy
Women should avoid dynamic breathing exercises during pregnancy, especially those that can lead to hyperventilation. This can affect the oxygen content in the blood and endanger the unborn child.

### Epilepsy
Dynamic breathing exercises can trigger or intensify epileptic seizures in some people.

### Mental Illnesses
People in unstable phases of life, as well as those with severe mental illnesses such as schizophrenia or acute panic attacks, should avoid dynamic breathing exercises as they can aggravate their mental condition.

*It is always advisable to consult a doctor before starting a new breathing exercise programme if you suffer from an illness or symptoms. Professional and experienced guidance in small groups is also recommended.*


## Everyday Tips

**Nasal Breathing**

If all you take away from this book is this single message, then I will be more than happy and satisfied: „**Breathe through your nose, breathe slowly, gently and silently.**"

Many people breathe almost exclusively through their mouth. This has many disadvantages. Mouth breathing is stress breathing, which stimulates the sympathetic nervous system, the stress mode in our nervous system. The brain does not differentiate between good and bad stress - stress is stress.

To tie in with nasal breathing: this is fundamentally important for activating our relaxation system and getting off the stress hamster wheel that causes illness.

Practise this in as many life situations as possible. When walking, hiking, jogging, doing sport - in every activity. Practise it when you sleep by covering your mouth. YES, you heard right. The nose is an organ that can be trained.

Balanced physical fitness, nutrition and an appropriate sleep rhythm favour your natural breathing.

To train your nervous system, there is really only one rule - regularity of use. This can be light, experimental and playful.

Simply try out my following tips and modify them to suit your own needs.

These habits promote your green area and are easy to integrate into your everyday life:

- Daily walks regardless of the weather, accompanied by consistent nose breathing. If the weather is rainy or damp, I recommend a warm shower and, if necessary, a warm cup of tea on your return.

- Cover your mouth to sleep - I'm amazed at the effect myself. The face becomes much more relaxed. Nasal breathing becomes even more natural in everyday life. No bad breath or dry mouth in the morning and less snoring.

- Gentle stretches. Make sure that you stay at the minimum stretch and wait for your breath to flow. Then listen to your body and slowly deepen the stretch. Start dancing with your breath and listen to the impulses that come from your body.

- Set yourself mobile phone, social media and TV restrictions and stick to them strictly. You can set yourself a timer and plan your time consistently. Example for people who use social media for work or leisure: 25 minutes of concentrated work. 5 minutes of conscious breathing, walking around, stretching, drinking tea, 25 minutes of publishing social media posts, 5 minutes break. Repeat.

- Switch off your computer for a certain time every evening and choose activities that calm your nervous system. Conversation, walking, eating, reading, meditation, bathing, candles, music and more.

- A regional, seasonal diet is essential. Check and, if necessary, reduce the volume of food you eat and try to bring the food into your mouth as you exhale.

- Chew thoroughly before swallowing. This will slow down your food intake. You will feel better when you are full.

- Nasal breathing and natural breathing are often made more difficult by the wrong food. Avoid sugar and other mucus-forming foods such as dairy products and cereals containing gluten as much as possible. This will clog your intestines, nasal passages and lungs.

- Have your blood tested periodically (every 3-6 months), look at your inflammation levels. Choose appropriate dietary supplements or natural medicines that can significantly support your body in finding its balance again.

  There are many herbal formulas to bring the body into balance, that strengthen your immune system, promote detoxification, reduce phlegm disease and strengthen your lungs, among other things. Take advantage of the support of trained therapists and doctors to optimise your system.

## Values - A Path to Inner Peace

Many people long for a deeper meaning and sustainable values that enrich and fulfil our lives.

Our true values, those inner guiding stars, can give you support in difficult times and show you the way. By focussing on your breath and connecting with your inner self, you can get in touch with your deepest beliefs and gain clarity about your priorities.

Initially, we often choose words that we have inherited from our parents or society. However, until we really feel them and fill them with our experiences, they are nothing more than empty word shells.

Non-violent communication, a powerful method of interpersonal connection, can support you in expressing your values authentically and resolving conflicts in a respectful way. By listening empathetically and expressing your needs, you can create an atmosphere of understanding and acceptance that enables you to act in accordance with your values.

This guide is a journey to your innermost beliefs, which you can put into practice with the help of VAGUS FLOW®.

It encourages you to go your own way and let your inner compass guide you, even if that means swimming against the current.

By consciously connecting with your values and integrating them into your daily life, you can find inner peace. Because when you act in harmony with yourself, you can lead a life that corresponds to your true self and fulfils you with joy and meaning.

# Non-Violent Communication

In this section, you will learn how to describe your inner perceptions and experiences in a flowery, rich and nuanced way. The use of multiple adjectives is a powerful tool to express your feelings and thoughts and to connect with yourself and others. By consciously enriching your language with an abundance of adjectives, you can express your feelings in a more nuanced way and encourage clearer communication. Practise this in conversations with other people. The aim is to communicate your emotions and perceptions honestly.

## Exercise

For a practical application of what you have learnt, I recommend the following exercise:

Sit or lie down comfortably. Choose a suitable word from the following list of adjectives and repeat it a few times internally, like a mantra. Observe what happens to your breath, your body and your mood. This can help you to connect with the different sensations and associations of the chosen word and deepen your self-awareness. Experiment with different words and observe how your reactions and sensations change.

The list comes from
**„1 Lists for non-violent communication, K. J. Becker, Seefeld"**

## Non-violent communication

adventurous
affectionate
alert
amazed
amused
appreciation
assured
attentive
authentic
awake
balanced
benevolent
blissful
calm
carefree
centred
cheerful
cheering
clear
close
collected
comforted
compassionate
concentrated
confident
connected
contented
cosy
courageous
creative lively

curious
delighted
determined
devoted
eagerly
easy
ecstatic
elated
electrified
enamoured
enchanted
encouraged
energetic
energised
enlivened
enriched
enthusiastic
excited
expectant
fascinated
feeling
filled with love
flourishing
free
friendly
fulfilled
full
full of admiration
funny
gentle

good-humoured
grateful
happy
harmonious
have desire
helpful
honest
hopeful
inspired
interested
intoxicated
involved
jubilant
liberated
light
lively
love of life
loving
marvelling
motivated
moved
open-minded
open-hearted
optimistic calm
overjoyed
passionate
peaceful
pleasantly
powerful
protected

proud
quiet
radiant
refreshed
relaxed
relieved
rested
reverent
satisfied
self-confident
sober
soothed
spellbound
stimulated
stirred
strong
sympathetic
tender
tense
touched
tranquil
trustful
trusting
unconcerned
upbeat
warm-hearted
warmly
well-mannered
well
wide awake

## Exercise: Sensing Values

Implementing the following exercise can take several weeks or even months. But it is worth the effort, because the result is fascinating and life-changing.

Write down a list of 20 words that are close to you. This is just a small example, as the list of possible words is long: authentic, compassionate, honest, respectful, generous, responsible, mindful, peaceful, just, loving, integrity, courageous, grateful. Go through them successively after the previous exercise, feeling the effect of the words on your breath, your body and your mood as you repeat them inwardly.

Reduce the list until there are only 5 essential words on it - your most important values. The values that you stand for and are passionate about.

The next step is to apply these values in all areas of your life and constantly check how and when you are not being completely true to yourself. Low moods and energy blockages are often an indicator that you are not being 100% true to yourself.

## Exercise: Silent VAGUS Moment

The „Silent VAGUS Moment" is an essential exercise that aims to facilitate deep rest and relaxation for body, mind and soul. It serves as a powerful conclusion to an active routine or as a stand-alone technique for stress reduction and inner contemplation.

### Execution

**Position:** Lie flat on your back on a comfortable surface. Your legs are slightly open and your arms are relaxed next to your body with your palms facing upwards. Close your eyes to focus your attention inwards.

**Breath and Relaxation:** Breathe in and out calmly. Let go of any tension with each exhalation. Guide your attention through your body and allow each part to relax further.

**Mental Calming:** Use this time to release thoughts and worries. Allow yourself to be fully in the here and now in these moments, free from any stress or pressure.

**Reflection and Renewal:** Use the silence to reflect on your current life circumstances, joys and challenges. Ask yourself the question: „What would I regret most if I had to die now?" Let this reflection become a source of clarity that shows you what needs to change in your life.

**Deepening:** The „Silent VAGUS Moment" not only offers the opportunity for physical and mental relaxation, but also for self-reflection. This practice encourages you to evaluate the current state of your life in order to be true to your values and desires. By regularly engaging in this exercise, you can sustainably increase your quality of life and inner satisfaction and actively realise the changes you want to make in your life.

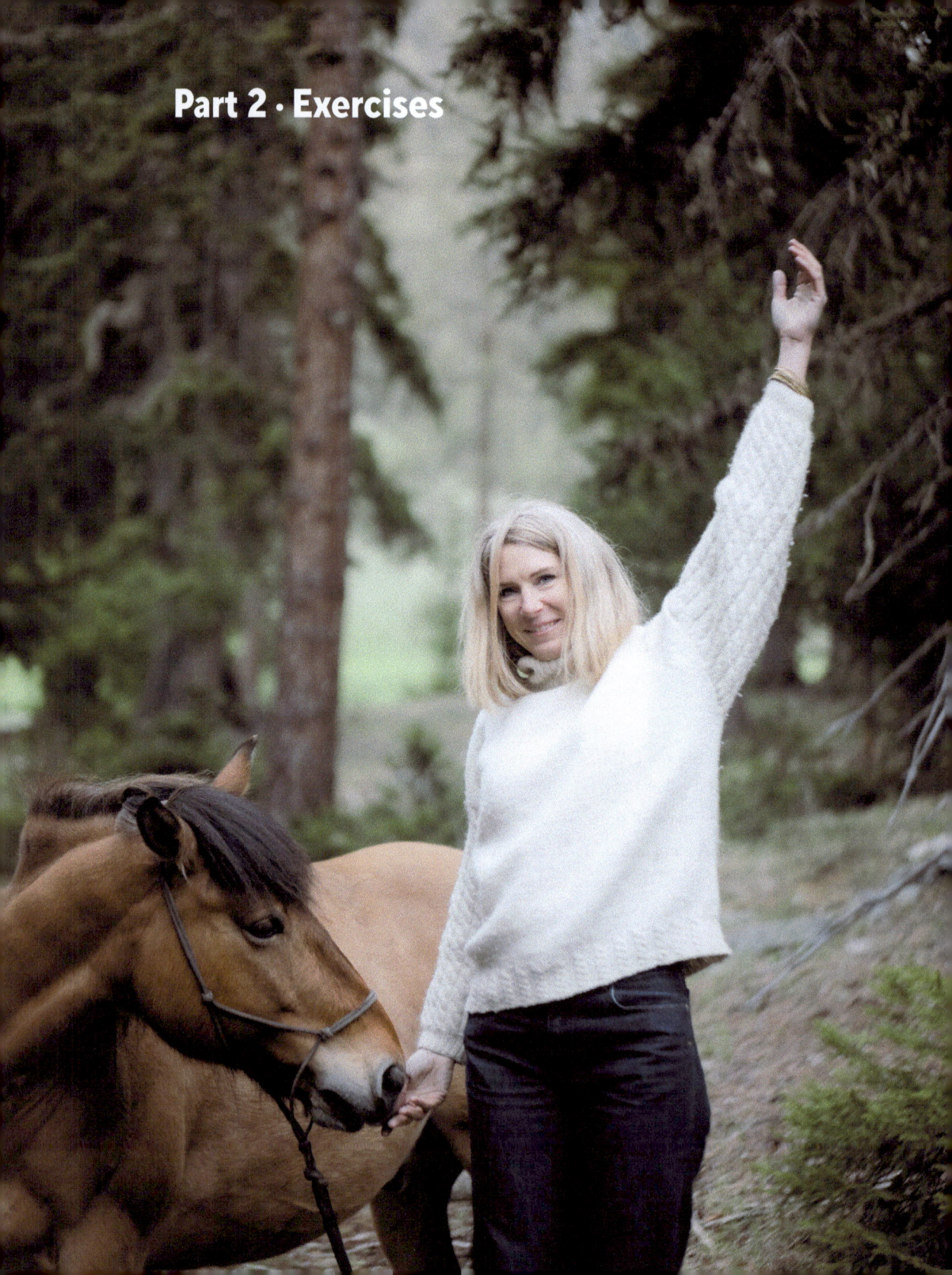

# From a Companion and Friend

About six years ago, in the magical, dreamy atmosphere of Guarda, I met a remarkable woman called Christina who, as a horse whisperer, filled her life with a unique vitality and alertness.

Christina's calm charisma and vibrant presence immediately captivated me. She is a source of inspiration that invites you to freely develop and realise your own ideas. With her ability to continuously create something new, she opens up spaces for innovation and creativity.

In recent years, Christina and I have travelled a similar path and have been able to enrich each other in many ways. Whether it was literature, financial knowledge, personal growth or our individual development, Christina always proved to be a valuable companion.

Her foresight and clairvoyance testify to a deep insight into human nature. Christina is empathetic and makes everyone feel heard and valued. When she enters a room, it is illuminated and she has the ability to guide and support people on their path. It is a real pleasure to spend time with Christina, be it just for a day or just a few hours. I sincerely hope that she can experience her fullness and freedom in everything she does.

Christina has her heart in the right place and enriches every place and every encounter with her presence. It is no coincidence that I have her in my life and in my immediate environment. We both owe our resonance with each other to our openness to life.

*Best regards, Renato Marni*
*Author, 18-time Taekwon-do world champion and 28-time world champion maker*

**Steps**

„As every blossom fades
and all youth sinks into old age,
so every life's design, each flower of wisdom,
attains its prime and cannot last forever.
The heart must submit itself courageously
to life's call without a hint of grief,
A magic dwells in each beginning,
protecting us, telling us how to live.

High purposed we shall traverse realm on realm,
cleaving to none as to a home,
the world of spirit wishes not to fetter us
but raise us higher, step by step.
Scarce in some safe accustomed sphere of life
have we establish a house, then we grow lax;
only he who is ready to journey forth
can throw old habits off.

Maybe death's hour too will send us out new-born
towards undreamed-lands,
maybe life's call to us will never find an end
Courage my heart, take leave and fare thee well."

*Hermann Hesse*

In this 2nd part of the book, we focus on the practical application of various exercises, divided into three categories:
- **Empathic-Breath**
- **Detox-Breath**
- **Gentle-Breath**

Breathing techniques, physical exercises and awareness practices are designed to support you in putting theory into practice and integrating it into your everyday life. Learn how to use your breath as a compass for your self-assessment and how to choose the right intervention for the moment.

Dancing, singing, tapping your body, massaging your hands, shaking, trembling and other activities are important for strengthening your body awareness and releasing stress.

**Please note and reflect on the following after each exercise:**

- How do you feel? Before, during and after?

- Describe this in concrete physical terms and use as many adjectives from the Nonviolent Communication list (page 81) as possible.

- What is your mood like?

Have fun practising and putting it into practice.

You can find the exercises filmed by Christina Koller in the shop at **www.sanajer.ch** – online breathing course

# EMPATHIC BREATH

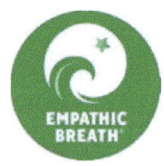

In the green area, the feeling of joy, security and well-being in social interaction is decisive. This means that you should particularly promote small moments of happiness and joy.

Bear in mind that for many people this is like having to learn a new language, as they have to learn how to rest, how to be, how to nurture joy. The feeling of being calm has not been sufficiently learnt.

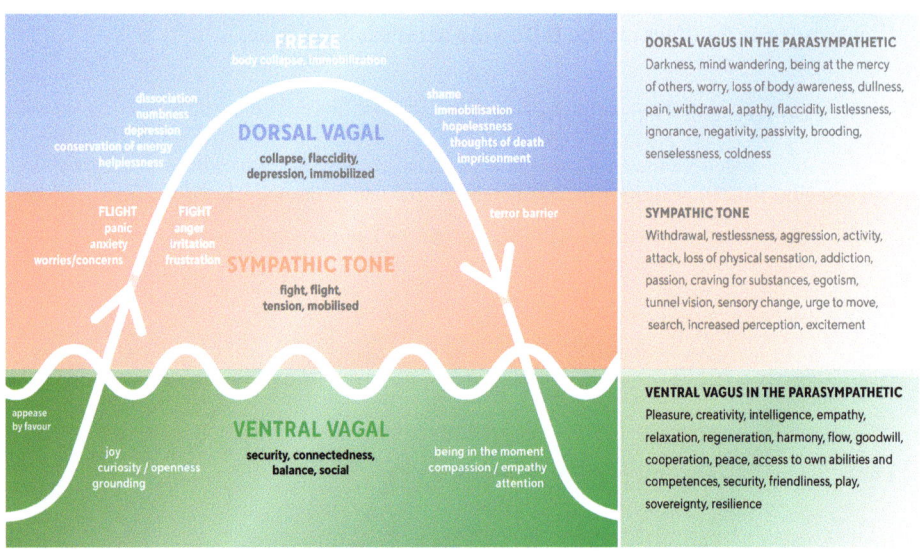

VAGUS FLOW© Theory · 2023

It is important to promote and strengthen the **ventral vagal** state as often as possible. Access to our sustainable performance, creativity and potential is only possible in this state, mixed with a pinch of sympathetic nervous system. We can also feel empathy, as this region of the brain is switched off when stress levels rise.

When you feel these characteristics, you experience a great sense of happiness.

## 1. Breath Awareness

Let's start with the most basic and most important exercise - developing your breath awareness.

**Integration into daily life:** To encourage ongoing breath awareness, it is helpful to use everyday objects or habits as memory anchors. This could be a special piece of jewellery, a motivating sticker, a certain melody, regular alarm clock signals or similar. Every time your attention is drawn to these anchors - whether by sight or sound - take a moment to observe your breath. Pay attention to how your breath is flowing, how your body feels and what emotional state you are in. This can be done in any posture and during any activity.

**I personally have the following anchors:** My finger ring, stickers on my computer and on my front door. I also set myself a timer every 25-45 minutes if I spend days or weeks sitting in front of the computer for hours. I take moving breaks of 5-10 minutes or more.

**Attention practice:** Choose a comfortable position, whether sitting, standing or lying down. Give your breath time and space. Observe how and where in the body the breath is particularly present. Try to intervene as little as possible. Accept the present moment as it is.

**The effect of mindfulness:** What changes when you consciously give your breath space and follow it attentively? Observe the changes without judgement.

**Conclusion of the exercise:** Repeat this mindful observation over a few breathing cycles. When you are ready, let the exercise come to an end. Note that the breathing practice is not about effort, but about a light, carefree awareness.

## 2. Spaces of the Breath

This exercise invites you to explore the different spaces of your breath and to consciously perceive its influence on your body.

**Preparation:** Find a comfortable position, either sitting or lying down. Make sure your upper body is upright and relaxed to give your lungs and diaphragm the freedom to unfold.

**The journey begins:** Firstly, concentrate on the natural flow of air through your nose. Feel how it flows in and out, without any effort.

**The world of the chest:** Place your hands on your chest area, the tips of your fingers lightly touching your collarbones. With each breath, feel how your hands are gently raised and lowered. Let your attention sink into your chest. Observe the movement of your breath - the gentle expansion with each inhalation and the retraction with each exhalation. Notice which thoughts, feelings and emotions are released by the movement in your chest.

**Without influence:** Allow yourself to simply be an observer of your breath without the urge to control or change it.

**Discovering the abdomen:** Now place your hands on your abdomen and remain in a state of attentive observation. Feel the natural expansion with the inhalation and the retraction with the exhalation. What inner movements are awakened by the breath in your abdomen?

This exercise promotes understanding and awareness of your breath in different parts of the body. It teaches you to observe and experience the breath without intervening - an essential step on the path to inner peace and balance.

This is a way to connect with your body by learning to breathe consciously into individual parts of your body.

**Starting position:** Find a comfortable sitting or lying position that allows you to concentrate fully on the exercise.

**Focus on your right hand:** Visualise your breath flowing directly into your hand as if it were an integral part of your right lung. You may visualise a pulsating light that illuminates and energises the hand from the inside with every breath.

**Intensify your perception:** Pay attention to the sensations in your hand. Does it start to tingle or pulsate? Does it feel warmer? Observe every sensation, be it flowing, warmth, cold or even pain. Breath and attention can reveal previously unnoticed tensions. If you give these sensations space and accept them without resistance, tensions can be released.

**Integration and awareness:** At the end of the exercise, expand your focus to both hands. Feel the possible difference between the left and right hand. What feeling does this perception trigger?

**Exercise outlook:** You can apply this technique to any part of your body. Especially in stressful situations or in moments of emotional stress, this application offers a valuable resource to avoid being drawn into thought loops or emotional whirlpools.

This exercise sharpens your inner perception and promotes the connection between breath and body awareness.

Start with a simple yet profound exercise - breath observation. This is a tool to help you connect with the subtle yet powerful energy of your breath.

**First step: Time and space for your breath**
Find a comfortable position. Give yourself and your breath time and space. Observe how your breath flows and in which area of your body you feel it most strongly. Don't try to consciously control or change it. Allow yourself to simply be in the now, with everything that is.

**Ask yourself:** What changes when I give my breath space and consciously recognise it?

**Second step: Inspiring words**
Browse through the list of adjectives used in non-violent communication and be inspired by their diversity. Choose a word that resonates and replay it quietly in your mind.
Observe what movements it evokes in you - in your body, in your feelings and how it affects your breathing. Feel the changes that each word causes and explore the unique meaning it has for you, your body and your breath. With practice, you will learn to recognise and appreciate the subtle differences.

**Third step: Diverse perception**
Describe your observations to yourself in as much detail and diversity as possible. Use your entire vocabulary to describe the physical sensations, the thoughts that pass through and the feelings and emotions that arise. Allow yourself to describe these elements of your experience in a variety of words, be they pragmatic or poetic. Repeat this breath observation over several cycles. Let the exercise end in stillness and silence.

**Final thought**
It is important to approach this breathing practice without haste. Your breath should flow naturally and without effort. This exercise is an invitation to get to know yourself better and to fill word shells with meaning.

## 5. The Magic Finger Breathing

Take a moment to make yourself comfortable and close your eyes. Allow yourself to observe your breath in silence, let it flow freely and become aware of your current state of being.

- Now begin by gently bringing the tips of the fingers of both hands together. Hold them together for a few breaths and feel: What effect does this simple gesture have on your breathing rhythm, on your physical sensations?

- Open your hands and bring your thumbs and index fingers into contact. Notice how your breathing pattern and physical sensations change.

- Next, open your hands again and bring your ring finger and little finger together. Go through the exercise again.

- Open your hands and only touch with your middle fingers. Return to the observation.

- Return to the starting point by bringing all fingers together again.

- Then repeat the whole process.

- Now position the palm of your left hand facing upwards and gently place the palm of your right hand on top of it. Fold your hands. What happens at this moment?

As with all forms of breath and body observation, there is no right or wrong. Your personal experience is paramount and it is always valid, even if it differs from the experience of many others.

The fascinating thing about this exercise is that for many people, even minimal changes in the touch of the fingers can bring about an adjustment in the breathing pattern. Often a change in emotional state is also perceived in the process.

**Back to the Roots of the Art of Breathing**

Cultivating natural breathing in daily life means becoming aware of the quality of our breath: Inhaling through the nose, carried by the diaphragm, gently, quietly, slowly and rhythmically. The exhalation is relaxed, while the abdomen vibrates in harmony with each breath.

This type of breathing forms the foundation of all further breathing exercises and techniques and is considered an essential practice. It not only supports sporting activities, walks and hikes through efficient oxygen utilisation and reduced acidification of the body, but also activates our relaxation system.

To approach this natural breathing, start by taking a comfortable position and relaxing.

- Place one hand on your chest and the other on your upper abdominal area so that the palm is between the top of your sternum and your belly button.

- Pay attention to the hand on your chest first. Feel how your breath lifts the hand and your chest like a wave. Observe whether there is any movement or whether the chest remains still. Remain in this observation for a few breaths.

- Then shift your attention to the lower breathing space. Feel how your abdominal wall expands with each inhalation and sinks back towards your spine with the exhalation. Allow yourself to be carried by this movement for a few breaths. Now be aware of both breathing zones simultaneously for a few breaths.

- Now focus on leaving the chest area as still as possible so that all the breathing activity comes from the abdomen. The chest remains still while the abdominal wall rises and falls rhythmically.

- Relax into the exhalation and let go as if each exhalation is a short pause, a brief moment of rest. The inhalation follows naturally.

The more you relax into this flow of breath, the softer and slower your breathing becomes. Stay in this natural breathing pattern for a few minutes.

## 7. Breathing Spaces

### A Journey through the Body

Make yourself comfortable in a quiet place, sitting or lying down.

- Begin this journey of discovery by placing both hands on your chest, with your fingertips lightly touching your collarbones. Feel how your chest expands when you inhale and relaxes again when you exhale. You can feel how your bones and collarbones expand slightly and how your tissue is stretched and massaged with every breath.

- Then move your hands to the sides of your ribs. Let your attention follow the movement of your ribs. They open with each inhalation and close again with the exhalation. Feel the dynamic expansion and the calming contraction.

- Then place your hands on your abdomen. Observe how your abdomen expands as you inhale and contracts as you exhale. It is as if you are inviting life in and releasing it with every breath, in a natural, calming rhythm.

It is always a fascinating experience to recognise how the body is moved, massaged, kneaded and stretched with every breath. This exercise is an invitation to explore and appreciate the wonders of your own body.

Take as much time as feels right for you and practise with ease, without effort and with gen-tleness. Let yourself be guided by the natural intelligence of your breath and enjoy the deep connection to yourself.

**An Anchor in Everyday Life**

- Wherever you are, whether standing, sitting or moving, and whatever you are doing, take a moment to pause and observe your breath.

- Feel which areas of your body the breath flows into. Which breathing space seems to be moving the most? What is the rhythm of your breath at this moment? Use as many descriptive words as possible to capture your sensations and try to leave any judgement aside. Just be an observer of what is, without any idea of how your breath should be.

- Allow yourself to accept what is happening and let go of all expectations of your breath. Repeat this exercise for several breaths and integrate it into your routine again and again throughout the day. The more often you incorporate this into your daily routine, the more natural your awareness of your breath will become.

**Over time, this regular breath observation can become an integral part of your life, similar to everyday habits such as brushing your teeth or tying your shoes. It is important because it subtly makes your life easier and more mindful and meditation becomes possible in every moment. Use the graph of the wave to assess yourself.**

**A Window into your Inner World**

Find a quiet place where you can sit down comfortably and keep a notebook to hand.

• Start by closing your eyes and directing your attention to your breath. What is happening inside you right now? Take a moment to explore what's going on inside you as you observe your breath coming in and out through your nose.

• Place your hands on your chest and feel the movements and rhythm of your breath and body. Then move your hands to your belly and allow yourself to feel the subtle movements there that follow your breath.

• Change the position of your hands to your ribs. Here too, feel the movements and rhythm created by your breath and body.

• Finally, place your hands on your thighs and use the lip brake to exhale a few times through your pursed lips with pleasure and without making a sound. Breathe in through your nose.

• Release this and feel what has changed.

Now is the time to reflect on your experience. Take out your notebook and answer the following questions. Write your answers using as many descriptive adjectives as possible to accurately capture the experience:

How is my breath flowing?
How does my body feel?
What is my mood like?
What were my most remarkable experiences during this exercise?

Reflection not only helps you to become more aware of your breath and your body, but also to immerse yourself in your personal experience and consciously explore it. It offers you the opportunity to make a connection between your physical and emotional state and to gain insights that often go unnoticed in everyday life.

**Creating Awareness in Everyday Life**

You can integrate conscious nasal breathing into any everyday situation: When walking, exercising, talking and even when eating.

When talking, make sure that you speak while exhaling, then pause briefly, inhale and only continue your speech with the next exhalation.

It's similar with eating: Feed yourself food while you exhale, chew consciously and take your time to breathe, slowly and with relish.

When walking or exercising, breathe exclusively through your nose to maximise the efficiency and cleansing of your airways.

To prepare your nasal awareness, find a comfortable position, whether standing or sitting.

• Begin to observe the flow of air through your nose. Visualise the air flowing in like a silver thread, quietly making its way to the bottom of the pelvis and rising back up as you exhale. Repeat this for a few breaths and notice the effects on your breath, your body and your mood.

Incorporate this into your day as often as possible. Set yourself little reminders, be it through alarm clocks, notes or objects, until this way of breathing has become second nature. Nasal breathing helps to calm your mind, relax your body and improve your general well-being.

**The Nocturnal Exercise**

Sleep is an integral part of nasal breathing. Ideally, you should breathe through your nose around the clock, 24/7. Like any other organ, the nose needs to be used regularly. The principle of „use it or lose it" applies here - a less-used nose can lose its function and, in the worst case, even constrict.

A special experiment is coming up to support your nasal breathing at night: Get some medical tape from the pharmacy or drugstore. Choose a tape that is elastic and gentle on the skin to avoid injuring your lips. The experiment involves taping your mouth shut at night. This method prevents the mouth from drying out during sleep, ensures that the air you breathe is warmed and filtered, promotes relaxation in the facial area, supports deeper sleep and can reduce snoring. This practice can even reduce morning bad breath.

Even if the idea may seem unusual at first, it is worth the experience. Sometimes we can embrace new methods in order to feel their effect on us.

## Personal Experience

„For years I was a woman of action. Constantly on the move, jumping from one activity to the next, always looking for the next adrenaline rush. It seemed as if stillness and inactivity were my greatest enemies.

But then, one day, I began my training as a breathing therapist. This step opened up a whole new world to me: the world of conscious breathing. Suddenly, pausing was no longer a sign of weakness, but a source of strength. I learnt to be with myself, to stay in the moment and embrace my emotions.

I found this difficult at first. The exercises I was taught seemed boring and slow, even uninteresting. How could mere breathing be comparable to the rush of fast movement and constant activity? But over time, as I learnt the patience to endure myself and appreciate stillness, I began to understand. Conscious breathing brought about a profound change in my life. It was as if I had discovered a hidden treasure within me that was just waiting to be brought to light.

Through breathing therapy, I not only found myself, but also a deeper, more fulfilling sense of existence. It was as if I had only scratched the surface all those years and had now finally found my way into the depths."

*Christina Koller*

# DETOX BREATH

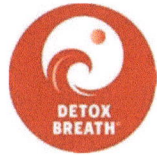

**In the red zone, the feelings of anger, restlessness, fear, as well as fight and flight as actions are central.**

In the sympathicotonic state, inhalation and mouth breathing are favoured. Therefore the interventions in Detox Breath are more dynamic. They are aimed at exhalation, regaining body awareness and letting off steam, without going beyond your limits and exhausting yourself in the process.

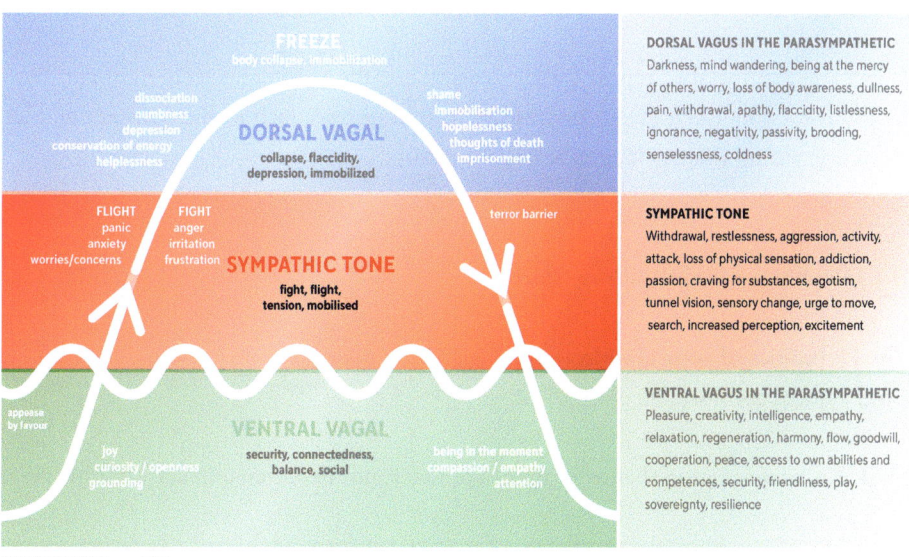

VAGUS FLOW© Theory · 2023

## 12. A Releasing Breath

### The Art of Letting Go
Make yourself comfortable in a quiet place, whether sitting or lying down.

- Breathe in as slowly and as fully as it feels right for you. Fill yourself with the breath, let it expand your space. Then hold the breath for a moment, for exactly as long as it feels comfortable and beneficial.

- As you exhale, let the breath out slowly, smoothly and without noise. To intensify this process, shape your lips as if you were blowing a low whistle. This is the lip brake technique, which further slows down your breathing flow and helps you slide into relaxation.

- Surrender to the exhalation and feel it. Remain still and attentive until the inhalation starts again of its own accord. Let the air flow in naturally through your nose.

If you feel comfortable, repeat these releasing breaths as often as feels right and harmonious for you. Each breath invites you to immerse yourself in the moment and let go of everything that no longer belongs to you.

## 13. Diaphragm Mobilisation - Part 1

### The Dynamics of your Diaphragm
Find a quiet, comfortable place to sit.

- Begin by massaging the lower tip of your sternum to soften and activate this area.

- Then position your fingers in the centre of the lower ribs, ready to connect with your breath.

- Inhale, filling your lungs completely with air.

- As you exhale, gently lean forwards and curl up, running your fingers gently under your ribs as if you were initiating an internal embrace of your diaphragm.

- Hold your breath in this position to intensify the mobilisation.

- Sit upright again and inhale.

- Exhale and lean forwards again, sliding your fingers under your ribs. Hold your breath again to mobilise the diaphragm to the maximum.

- Sit up, inhale.

Repeat this exercise at your own pace as often as feels right for you. You can vary the position of your fingers slightly on each pass to massage different areas of your diaphragm and promote deep mobilisation and relaxation.

This exercise helps you to mobilise your diaphragm.

## 14. Diaphragm Mobilisation - Part 2

### Waves of Breath
Lie on your back. Give yourself a moment to arrive and connect with your natural flow of breath. Observe how your breath flows in and out and find your own rhythm.

- With each exhalation, let your lower back sink to the floor and feel the connection to the earth.

- As you inhale, roll your back into a hollow cross.

- Repeat this movement a few times, allowing your breath and the movements to flow into each other. Feel how your body and breath feel after each round.

- When you are ready to intensify the exercise, lift the pelvis on an inhalation and roll upwards vertebra by vertebra.

- With each exhalation, lower your back back down to the floor vertebra by vertebra.

Repeat this movement as often as feels right and comfortable for you. Once you have finished, stretch your legs out and feel for yourself.

This form of diaphragmatic mobilisation helps to improve the flexibility of your back, promotes more conscious breathing and strengthens the connection between your breath and your movements.

## 15. Diaphragmatic Breathing

### A Foundation of Calm
Sit down with your upper body naturally upright.

- Place one hand on your chest and the other on your abdomen, directly above your belly button.

- Close your eyes and allow yourself to sink into a state of calm. During this exercise, concentrate on keeping the upper hand still to ensure that all breathing activity comes from the lower breathing space - the diaphragm.

- Breathe in exclusively through your nose without straining. As you inhale, the abdominal cavity expands and the abdominal wall rises.

- Now exhale slowly, intensifying the exhalation by pulling the abdominal wall in as far as possible towards your spine at the end. Imagine a bellows forcing the air out of you. At the end of the exhalation, start the next inhalation without pausing.

- Breathe in, expanding your abdomen as if you were inflating a balloon in your stomach.

- Breathe out, pulling the abdominal wall inwards to push out as much air as possible.

Repeat this cycle for 3-5 almost silent diaphragmatic breaths. After this sequence, take a minute to feel the effects of the exercise. This tracking marks the end of the first round.

If you wish, you can repeat the exercise to further deepen and consolidate your ability to breathe diaphragmatically. This exercise helps to mobilise your diaphragm and strengthen your muscles.

## 16. Breathing under Stress - Regulation via Box Breathing

The box breathing exercise is a breathing technique designed to reduce stress and calm the mind. Sit in a comfortable position, either on a chair with an upright spine or on a cushion on the floor.

- Close your eyes and relax your shoulders.

- Breathe in through your nose and count slowly to four.

- Hold your breath and count slowly to four again.

- Breathe out and count to four again.

- Hold your breath again and count to four.

- Repeat this cycle several times, usually for 3-5 minutes, or for as long as it feels comfortable.

As you perform this breathing exercise, try to focus on the steady rhythm of your breath and let go of any distracting thoughts. This helps to calm the mind and reduce stress.

Vary the intervals. You can adjust them to your rhythm at any time. For example, inhale 4 times, pause 4 times, exhale 8 times, pause 4 times.

## 17. The Power of Breath

If you suffer from asthma, cardiovascular disease or panic attacks, or are pregnant, it is better not to do this exercise, or only with the utmost caution.

Sit or lie down comfortably.

- Take 10 big breaths. In through the nose and out through the nose or mouth. No pauses, so that a so-called circular or connected breath is created. After the last inhalation, let your breath flow out passively and remain in the breathing pause, silence, for as long as you feel comfortable.

If you like, you can repeat this for 2-3 rounds. Reflect and give yourself a moment's break before returning to your everyday life.

Many people love the effect of this exercise. It can induce a tingling sensation, a trance-like state or an intoxicating feeling of happiness. During the breaks, it can bring calm and tranquillity. However, many people feel unwell. Panic attacks, asthma attacks or other consequences, including fainting, can occur. If this occurs, exhale slowly through pursed lips, inhale quietly through the nose, the coachman's seat (round spine, lean forwards, elbows supported) can be helpful and support regulation. Kneading your hands, washing your face with cold water, shaking and patting can also help.

From a physiological point of view, this is hyperventilation. It brings the body's biochemistry into imbalance and reduces cerebral blood flow by up to 60 per cent within a very short time.

## A Step-by-Step Overview

Start by lying down on a comfortable surface. Make sure your back is flat on the floor and you feel comfortable.

Allow yourself to take a few natural breaths. With each breath, you should try to relax more and let go of inner tension.

- Tighten your legs and position your feet flat on the floor, about hip-width apart, directly in front of your buttocks, with your knees pointing upwards.

- On the next inhalation, slowly lift your pelvis off the floor by rolling your spine up bit by bit until you are in shoulder bridge. At the same time, move your arms synchronised over your head to the floor behind you.

- Exhale, hold your breath and then begin to slowly unroll your spine vertebra by vertebra during this short breathing pause until your pelvis touches the floor.

- With the next inhalation, lift your pelvis into a shoulder bridge while simultaneously placing your arms behind your head.

- Exhale and bring your arms back to the floor next to your body.

Repeat these movements a few times, making sure that your breathing and movements are synchronised.

After repeating this a few times, finish by stretching your legs out and lying flat on your back. Take a moment to reflect and savour the released tension in the diaphragm and the entire spine.

This exercise not only helps to loosen the diaphragm and deepen your breathing, but also has a strengthening effect.

**Overview:** DETOX Breath is an intensive breathing technique specifically designed to stimulate the vagus nerve and bring about a deep inner cleansing as well as an increase in energy and vitality. This technique promotes physical and mental clarity through dynamic inhalation and exhalation.

**You can find the fully guided drum meditation DETOX Breath in the shop at www.sanajer.ch.**

- **Preparation:** Take a comfortable sitting position and allow yourself to observe your natural breathing for a few moments in silence. Make sure you are in a healthy state, as DETOX Breath is not suitable for certain conditions such as asthma or cardiovascular disease.

- **Active breathing:** After a calm exhalation, start breathing rapidly and forcefully, expanding the abdomen with each inhalation and pulling forcefully towards the spine on the exhalation. Aim for a fast breathing rate of around 1-2 breaths per second, which produces a clear breathing sound.

- **Rhythm:** Perform this intensive breathing for about 20 cycles. After the last exhalation, hold your breath for as long as you feel comfortable before taking another deep breath and holding it again to intensify the effect.

- **Conclusion:** After one round, return to natural breathing and repeat as necessary. At the end, give yourself enough time to rest and integrate the activating effect of the exercise on your body and mind.

**Advanced practice:** For those who want to intensify this, rhythmic support through audio recordings can be helpful to synchronise the breathing.

**Special notes:** DETOX Breath is not only a method for strengthening physical and mental well-being, but also for promoting energetic cleansing. By consciously activating the vagus nerve, this exercise supports improved regulation of the autonomic nervous system. Knowing how to do it can also interrupt an acute panic attack. However, you should always be professionally supervised.

## 20. Diaphragm Training with Resistance

The following exercise is a final step in your breathing journey.

- Begin this exercise by wrapping a cloth around your ribs. The cloth acts as resistance and will help you to train your diaphragm more effectively.

- Pull the cloth together and take a breath. Feel how your ribs expand against the resistance of the cloth.

- As you exhale, pull the cloth together a little tighter to increase the resistance. Consciously breathe in against this resistance. This helps to strengthen your diaphragm and supports the development of healthy breathing behaviour.

- Repeat this process at your own pace and for as long as it feels right and comfortable for you.

- Finally, release the cloth with an inhalation and take a moment to feel the effects of the exercise.

At the end of this exercise block, it's time to reflect. Pick up your notebook and take a moment to observe your breath.

Answer the following questions and try to use as many descriptive adjectives as possible in your answers:

How does my breath flow?
How does my body feel?
What is my mood like?
What do I take away from this challenge in particular? What were my most remarkable experiences?

## 21. VAGUS FLOW® Reflection

Congratulations on your courage and perseverance in facing these exercises and yourself. If you wish, please feel free to share your feedback on your experiences. It is a great opportunity to look back on your journey and appreciate what you have achieved.

A guide to inner mindfulness.

Please have a notebook ready to write down your thoughts and feelings.

Find a comfortable sitting position.

Close your eyes and focus your attention on your breath. Consciously notice what is going on inside you at this moment.

• Breathe naturally a few times without trying to control your breath.

• Place one hand on your chest. Feel the movements and rhythm of your breath and the associated changes in your chest.

• Then position one hand on your stomach. Be aware of the movements and rhythm of your breath and abdomen.

- Now practise diaphragmatic breathing, in which the chest remains largely motionless and the movement is mainly felt in the abdominal area. Repeat this way of breathing a few times.

- Intensify abdominal breathing. Pull your abdomen towards your spine as you exhale and contract it more strongly at the end of the exhalation, as if you want to push the air out.

- Place your hands on your thighs and let the breath out a few times while humming.

Slowly disengage from the exercise and take a moment to feel and experience the effect.

Take your notebook and reflect on the following questions. Try to describe your answers with as many adjectives as possible:

What are my main goals for today?
How can I enhance my focus and concentration?
What positive habits can I develop to improve my well-being?
How can I effectively manage stress in challenging situations?

This reflection exercise offers you the opportunity to gain insights into your inner state and to consciously explore and document your experiences.

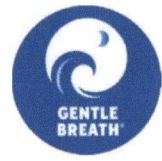

# GENTLE BREATH

In the blue area, the feelings of sadness, numbness, being beside oneself and being separated from the body are dominant.

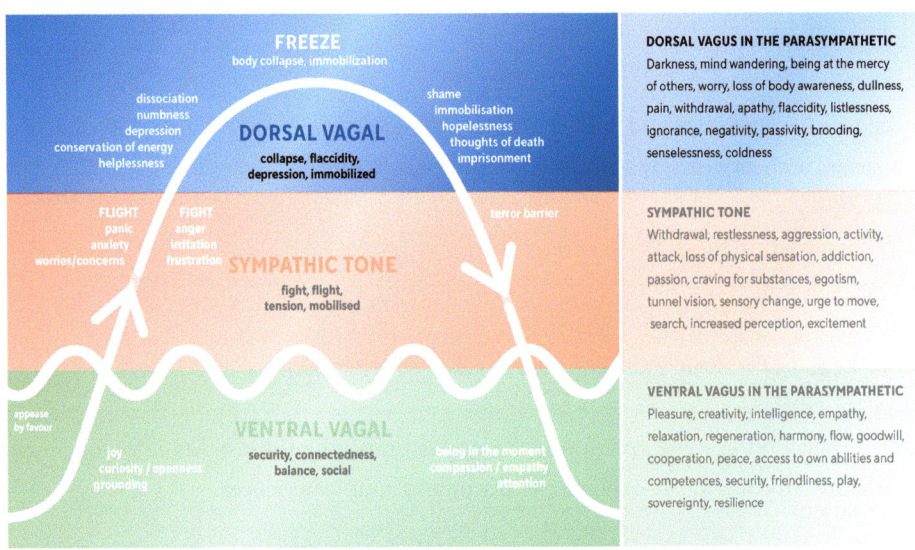

VAGUS FLOW© Theory · 2023

**In the dorsal vagal state** we are frozen, movement and exit can be tough and difficult because we are mentally immobile. That's why this chapter is called GENTLE BREATH: „To be gentle" means to be gentle, loving and mindful of yourself. These qualities are particularly important when you find yourself in a rigid, depressive or physically restricted situation. Beginning with the mental activation of the mobile cortex, continuing with physical movement in order to find our way back to a mobile form and awaken from the state of freeze. These interventions can support us considerably during illness and convalescence and activate our inner healing powers.

It is particularly important to get off your thought carousel by consistently focussing on your breathing and body awareness. You can reflect on your problems and issues again later when you have gained a foothold in the constructive green area.

## 22. Gentle Breath

In the blue zone, the breath tends to be in the throat or is barely noticeable. This can be changed with the following 2 steps:

- The first step to get out of this state is to feel and accept that I don't feel anything.

- The second step is to pay attention to the breath and welcome it into the throat.

Breath is like water. It will always find its way. The important thing is to give it space and not restrict it. Observe what happens, notice the smallest changes and register the return of the body sensation.

## 23. Relax with the Exhalation

Find a comfortable position, whether sitting or lying down, and allow yourself to calm down. Take a moment to notice your breath - just observe it without intervening.

- Feel how your body rises and falls slightly with each breath. Let your breath flow freely and freely, don't try to control or direct it.

- Pay attention to both the inhalation and the exhalation. And then, with each exhalation, allow yourself to relax, to let go a little more.

- The inhalation will follow naturally without you having to exert yourself. After each inhalation, simply let go.

- Imagine that each exhalation is accompanied by a feeling of coming home. The exhalation is followed by a short pause, a moment of stillness, before the cycle begins again with the next inhalation.

Linger in this process and let the rhythm of your breath carry you along. Every breath is like a little journey. Feel how a deeper level of relaxation becomes possible with every exhalation, a gentle return to yourself.

## 24. VAGUS FLOW® Massage - Part 1

### Touching the Heart

Make yourself comfortable, sitting or lying down.

- Begin by placing your hands on your heart. Imagine how you take your heart in your hands and from this moment on, every touch is a caress with heart. Support the effect of your massage by observing your breath and connecting each touch with an inner relaxation.

- Run the fingertips of your right hand over your forehead, along your temple, over your cheek, down your neck to your collarbone. Let each movement flow into the next.

- Then change sides and repeat the strokes with the left hand - from the forehead, over the temple and cheek, down the neck to the collarbone. Find your own rhythm and repeat these movements mindfully.

- Your hands meet in the centre of your forehead. Sweep your fingers over your eyebrows, towards the corners of your eyes, under your eyes and then up the sides of your nose, back to your eyebrows.

- With each repetition, make the circles your fingertips draw a little larger. Touch the hairline, temples and cheekbones.

- Now run your fingers in small circles over your temples. Continue this calming movement and then move your fingers in circles over your temporomandibular joint.

- Pay particular attention to your jaw joint and massage it. Experiment with different levels of pressure and forms of movement to feel what works for you.

- Now massage your lower jaw, explore the tissue by pinching it and feel how it feels for you.

When you release yourself from the massage, pause for a moment and reflect. Notice how this VAGUS FLOW® massage makes your body and mind feel.

## 25. Hum

### An Exercise for Mindfulness and Relaxation

Breathe gently and slowly. If you feel dizzy or light-headed, this is a sign of over-breathing. Then take a break and breathe even more gently.

Find a comfortable position, whether sitting or lying down, and close your eyes.

- Breathe in naturally, slowly and with full awareness. After inhaling, hold your breath briefly. Then let the breath out while humming. The slower and gentler you breathe out, the longer and more intense the vibration will be.

- After exhaling, wait a moment until the natural impulse to inhale arises of its own accord. There will be a natural pause before the next buzzing exhalation.

- Repeat this process for 3 to 5 breaths and then feel inside yourself. Feel the after-effects of the exercise in your body.

- If you like, you can do several rounds of this exercise.

- Experiment with different pitches when humming. Each frequency creates its own vibration in the body. Observe which pitch produces the most pleasant vibrations for you.

Stop the exercise when it feels right for you. Open your eyes, but give yourself enough time to prepare for the transition back into your everyday life.

This exercise helps to slow down your breathing and promotes mindfulness through vibration.

## 26. VAGUS FLOW® Massage - Part 2

This section is dedicated to touching and massaging various parts of the head and shoulders. My instructions are suggestions: Play and experiment with it, find your own form of massage.

Start by adopting a comfortable position, sitting or lying down.

- Gently place your hands on your heart. Visualise placing your heart in your hands and from now on perform every touch from the heart. Support the potential of your massage by following your breath and the loving touches of your heart, and by going into an inner state of relaxation.

- Gently run the fingertips of your right hand over your forehead, temples, cheek and neck, down to your collarbone. Now change hands and repeat the movement with your left hand, starting at the forehead and ending at the collarbone.

- Repeat these strokes in a rhythm that is comfortable for you.

- Your hands meet at your forehead. Let them glide slowly over your face to the jaw joint. Press on your jaw joint and move your fingers towards your ears.

- Now devote yourself to massaging your ears, starting with the auricles. Grasp your earlobes and gently pull them in different directions - downwards, backwards and upwards. Increase the area you grasp with each pass. Use your index fingers to massage the area under the earlobes. Take a moment to do this.

- Now find the muscle strands of the head-turning muscles that run diagonally under your earlobe to the collarbones. Knead these strands carefully. Repeat the massage several times.

- Turn to your neck and massage the areas to the left and right of the vertebral column with targeted movements

- Finally, massage your shoulders to release any tension.

Detach yourself from the exercise. Close your eyes, observe your natural flow of breath and feel inside yourself. Take time to savour the effect of the massage and explore the deep connection between breath, touch and relaxation.

A way to achieve targeted relaxation.

This technique can be used specifically to address and release pain and tension in certain areas of the body. Focus specifically on a painful area of your body.

Find a comfortable position, either sitting or lying down, and focus your full attention on your breath and the area of pain.

- Start with a natural inhalation. Imagine directing the air directly into the painful area as if you were breathing in right there.

- Hold your breath and let it focus on the painful area.

- Then exhale while humming, keeping your attention on the affected area. Visualise releasing the pain with the exhalation.

- Repeat the process as often as you feel comfortable: inhale, hold briefly and release the tension as you exhale.

- Experiment with different pitches when humming to find out which frequency has the most pleasant vibration and therefore the best effect on the painful area.

After several repetitions, take a moment to feel for yourself. Observe whether anything has changed in relation to the pain or tension.

Learn to use the combination of breathing technique and humming to specifically influence painful areas of the body and possibly experience relief as a result.

The VAGUS energy flow exercise is a precise method for activating and balancing the dynamic forces of the sympathetic nervous system (via sun breathing) and the parasympathetic nervous system (via moon breathing). This promotes an understanding of the balance between energy and relaxation, between doing and being.

## SUN ENERGY ACTIVATION (SYMPATHETIC NERVOUS SYSTEM)

- **Position:** Find a comfortable sitting position and breathe in a relaxed manner.

- **Execution:** Close the left nostril and breathe in through the right one to fill your body with energy in a pleasant way. Hold your breath for as long as it feels good.

- **Conclusion:** Let the breath flow out more slowly than it flowed in. This phase activates the right side and therefore the sympathetic nervous system, which stands for warmth and activity. Ideal for moments that require strength, energy, focus and concentration.

## LUNAR RELAXATION ACTIVATION (PARASYMPATHETIC NERVOUS SYSTEM)

- **Preparation:** Come to rest in the same sitting position.

- **Execution:** Now close the right nostril and breathe in through the left. This stimulates the left side and the parasympathetic nervous system, which is responsible for relaxation and letting go. After inhaling, feel inside yourself and decide whether you want to pause to breathe or let your breath flow freely.

- **Conclusion:** Exhale more slowly than you inhale and optionally tighten the abdominal wall at the end of the exhalation to release the breath completely.

**Integration and application:** Practise both breathing techniques for 2-10 minutes each, depending on your needs and well-being. The alternation between sun and moon energy flow supports the harmonious balance of the VAGUS nerve and enables a smooth transition between activity and rest. Concluding, release yourself from the exercise and take a moment to feel the effect in your body and mind.

You can also do just one of the two exercises, depending on your current need for either rest or activity.

## 29. VAGUS Balance Breathing

VAGUS Balance Breathing is a profound practice for harmonising and cleansing the energetic pathways that run through our body. By alternating breathing through the left and right nostrils, a fine balance is established between the activating sympathetic nervous system and the calming parasympathetic nervous system. This technique not only promotes deep relaxation, but also supports the optimal functioning of the vagus nerve.

- **Positioning:** Take a comfortable sitting position and allow yourself to calm down. Start with natural, calm breathing and visualise the air flowing through your nose like a silver thread.

- After a calm exhalation, close the right nostril with the thumb of your right hand and breathe in through the left. Imagine how your body fills with energy while your chest remains calm.

- After inhaling, change the closing position: use the ring finger to close the left nostril and open the right one to exhale in a relaxed manner.

- Breathe in through the right nostril, then change the closing position and breathe out through the left.

- Continue this alternation after each inhalation.

Practice time: Take 5 to 10 minutes to achieve a profound effect. End VAGUS Balance Breathing with an exhalation through the left nostril and then allow yourself a moment of rest in a sitting or lying position.

Extension for advanced practitioners: For those who already have experience with this technique, it is possible to intensify the exercise by closing one nostril completely and the other partially. This variation challenges and promotes inner calm and adaptability, especially in preparation for colder times or if you have a blocked nose. Learn to maintain natural breathing even under difficult conditions.

Additional benefits: VAGUS Balance Breathing is an excellent preparation for challenges such as cold periods. It promotes relaxed breathing even with a blocked nose, without drawing in air noisily, which could put additional strain on the airways and sinuses.

## 30. VAGUS Rhythmic Breathing

VAGUS Rhythmic Breathing refines the technique of VAGUS Balance Breathing by adding rhythmisation. This advanced exercise intensifies the harmonising effect on the vagus nerve and the balance between the sympathetic and parasympathetic nervous system. By lengthening the exhalation compared to the inhalation, a deeper level of relaxation and regeneration is achieved.

- **Preparation:** Start with the familiar VAGUS balance breathing, in which you breathe alternately through each nostril. Let your breathing be natural and flowing.

- **Rhythmisation:** After a few regular breaths, add rhythmisation by lengthening the exhalation time compared to the inhalation time. For example, one possible rhythmisation is to breathe in for 4 seconds and out for 8 seconds.

- Keep this within a relaxed framework and remember the principle of „effortless endeavour".

- **Integrating breathing pauses:** After a few rounds of rhythmised breathing, you can add breathing pauses. Hold the breath after the inhalation for a duration equal to the length of your inhalation.

- **Practice time and conclusion:** Dedicate 5-10 minutes to this exercise. End VAGUS Rhythm Breathing with a relaxing exhalation and allow yourself a moment of rest, either sitting or lying down.

- **Creative extensions:** You can integrate various elements to support rhythmisation: Count the breaths, use mantras, hum or sing. These creative elements can deepen and personalise the experience.

- **Additional benefits:** VAGUS Rhythm Breathing not only promotes a sense of calm and relaxation, but also supports physical and mental regeneration. Through conscious and rhythmised breathing, you strengthen your ability to maintain calmness and balance in everyday life.

## 31. VAGUS Clear Breath

This is a powerful breathing technique for internal cleansing and clearing the airways, which is aimed directly at optimising vagus nerve function. It is excellent for promoting mental clarity and supporting physical well-being by actively clearing the airways.

- **Preparation:** Take a comfortable sitting position and find inner peace. Make sure you feel healthy as this technique is not recommended for certain conditions such as asthma or cardiovascular disease.

- **Active exhalation:** Place your hands on your belly to feel the movement. Begin to increase the exhalation by actively pulling the abdominal wall inwards and upwards. Repeat this increased exhalation 5-10 times.

- **Breathing out in bursts:** A natural inhalation is followed by a series of rapid, burst-like exhalations through the nose, similar to blowing out a candle. The exhalation is actively controlled by drawing in the abdominal wall, while the inhalation is passive. Focus either on the nose or on the movement of the abdominal wall.

- **How to perform:** Repeat 30-60 of these exhalations, which we define as one round. At the end of a round, let the breaths slowly fade out and after the last exhalation, remain empty until a reflexive inhalation begins.

- **Conclusion and repetition:** After a short natural breathing phase, repeat the exercise for a total of approximately three rounds. Then allow yourself a moment of rest and relaxation.

- **Special notes:** The VAGUS clear breath is not only an exercise for clearing the airways, but also a method for strengthening physical and mental resilience. The special thing about this exercise is that it triggers stress and thus cancels out the body's own state of stress - a paradoxical intervention that we could simply call „combating stress with stress".

## 32. Breath Observation and VAGUS FLOW®

### An Integrative Relaxation Method

To begin, find a relaxed position in which you can sit or lie down and allow yourself to enter a state of natural breathing. Give yourself this moment to consciously notice your breath.

- Run the fingertips of your right hand over your forehead, temples, cheek and neck, down to your collarbone. Take time to consciously feel each touch and allow it to take effect. Then smoothly switch to the other side.

- Repeat the same process with your left hand, starting at the forehead and moving down to the collarbone, following your own rhythm.

- When your hands meet at the forehead, let them glide slowly over your face up to the jaw joint. Apply gentle pressure or stroking movements to the jaw joint and then move your fingers to the ears, massaging the pinnae.

- Grasp your earlobes, gently pull them down, back and up, and repeat this several times. With each repetition, you can try to grasp the edge of the ear a little further up.

- Use your index fingers to massage underneath the earlobes.

- Then massage the muscle cords of the head-turning muscles that run diagonally from below the earlobes to the front of the collarbones. Knead and massage these areas carefully.

- Now turn to your neck and massage the areas to the left and right of the spine.

- Massage your skull by pressing and moving over the bones in a circular motion.

- Reach for your hair roots by grasping larger tufts of hair (if the hair length allows) and pulling on them.

- Finish by massaging your shoulders to release any remaining tension.

Detach from the exercise, close your eyes and return to observing your natural breath.

Take a moment to reflect and explore the effect of the whole exercise on your body and mind.

# CONCLUSION

The journey we have undertaken together through the various breathing, body and awareness exercises can be the path to yourself, to self-discovery and inner growth.

However, it may also be that the gentle exercises have caused you more stress and defence. Every experience is individual and is characterised by personal history and experience. What you feel and experience is exactly right and makes sense.

These exercises can be a tool to promote your physical health and strengthen your muscles. They may also create a space to dive deep inside yourself and explore your emotions.

The regular practice of breath observation forms the foundation. You have learnt to listen to the rhythm of your breath and become aware of how you feel at different moments - before, during and after. You have learnt how important it is to take time to deepen your breathing and connect with your inner self.

The aim of the exercises is to reduce your unconscious stress, activate you and improve your emotional regulation. They give you the space to deal with your own feelings and needs. They show you that you have the ability to heal yourself and promote your own well-being if you take the time to listen to yourself and love yourself.

## Seminar Participants Had the Following Experiences

„The breathing exercises created a connection to my own pain and strengthened my self-love and compassion. This led to a deep compassion for my fellow human beings."
*Simone Gehrli*

„Through breath observation, the breath becomes more subtle and the chronic coughing irritation disappears. I was used to always manipulating my breath."
*Joe Taugwalder*

„I have learnt so much through silence, meditation, hypnosis and mental techniques, as well as through various coaching sessions. But if the breath remains in the old pattern, I don't fully come to myself. That was my realisation after my visit with you. Thank you!"
*Daniela Joss*

„I was looking for something that would relax my nervous system and support me in finding my inner home. Through your work I have received such a valuable gift, breathing. Especially through your way of being and the space you gave me, new things were able to emerge for me. I was able to get to know my breathing anew and have new experiences. It goes on and on. I hope everyone gets to know your wonderful work. For your knowledge and this wonderful „tool", breathing. Thank you! It is a gift that you bring this into the world! „
*Jana*

It is advisable to regularly schedule time for these exercises and integrate them into your everyday life. Start with small steps and increase slowly to achieve lasting changes. The regularity of breath observation should be particularly emphasised, as it is an important part of the exercises.

## Advice on Personal Support

It is crucial to realise that emotions can become overwhelming during your practice. In such moments, it is important to be accompanied by a trusted professional, be it an experienced therapist or a qualified trainer. They can help you to understand and process your emotions and turn them into positive, trusting experiences.

Talking to a trusted professional allows you to reflect on your experiences and adapt your exercises to your personal needs. In addition, the ANS measurement can show how your nervous system reacts to the interventions. This can be a valuable method to track your progress and support your healing process. By adapting the exercises and techniques to your individual needs, you can create a deeper connection to your inner self and activate your inner resources to holistically improve your well-being.

## Disclaimer

This book is intended as a guide for personal development and well-being and is not a substitute for professional medical advice or treatment. Although the exercises and techniques in this book can help to reduce stress, improve emotional regulation and promote overall wellbeing, we accept no liability for any potential harm or injury that may result from the application of the methods presented.

Please note that this book is not a substitute for a visit to a doctor, therapist or other medical professional. In the event of serious health problems or mental illness, it is essential to seek professional help and undergo appropriate medical treatment. If in doubt, we encourage you to consult a qualified specialist for individual advice and support.

# FINAL WORD

In this book, you have explored a wealth of knowledge and wisdom to help you stand on the solid ground of your own being and fill your life with joy.

May resilience become second nature and vitality resonate in your every step. You have learnt to consciously control your energy balance and to navigate between restraint and full power.

Through the art of breath observation, mindfulness and the ability to be fully present in the present moment, you now have the tools to calm the whirlwind of thoughts and understand your state on the wave of life. You have been given the tools to bring yourself back into balance and now know when action is required and when simply being is the more powerful response.

The breath, your faithful companion, is a source of guidance and strength. It is your most honest partner, always telling you the truth about yourself, as long as you are willing to listen and heed the quiet hints. I sincerely hope that you continue to strengthen the bonds with this powerful ally so that you can walk your path with serenity and clarity.

This book should not be the end, but a shining milestone on your personal journey of discovery. A beginning that inspires you to explore further, to grow and to fully realise the wonderful potential that lies within you. With every breath you consciously take, you remember your strength, your ability to change and how beautiful it is to simply be.

We are human beings, deeply social beings. Traumatic experiences do not happen in isolation in a vacuum - and neither does healing happen alone. It is in connection with others that we realise our greatest potential to overcome and grow. Therefore, have the courage to seek support and dialogue when the storms of life become too strong. Together, the path to healing is not only easier, but often more profound and enriching.

With this in mind, may your life be filled with inner strength, joy and an unshakeable belief in yourself. Walk your path courageously and with an open heart, because it belongs to you alone.

I look forward to your personal breathing story, your networking, your contact, your constructive feedback and your testimonial.

*From the heart*
*Christina*

# THANK YOU

THANK YOU to all my companions, friends, teachers, coaches and beings who have helped my project come to life - who believed in me even in the most difficult moments and gave me wind beneath my wings.

THANK YOU to all the supporting angels who are not mentioned by name, but who have just as big a place in my heart.

Renato Marni

Rita Fasel

Ingfried Hobert

Tatjana Hagen

Tasnia Tarana

Katja Meuli

Team „Bündner Kommunikationsmacher"

Till Akira and Luna Makena Koller

Gosia Orlicz

Andrea Merkel

Sandra Lüthi

# Sources

Breath mainly means: experiencing, observing, playing and experimenting.
Inspiration comes from awareness, depth and regularity.

These books have particularly inspired me to deepen my theoretical work:

| | |
|---|---|
| Gabor Maté | „When the body says no" |
| Stephen W. Porges | „Accessing the Healing Power of the Vagus Nerve" |
| Deb Dana | „Anchored" |
| | „Polyvagal Theory in Therapy" |
| Ralph Skuban | „Atmen – heilt – entspannt – zentriert" |
| | „Pranayama" |
| | „Die Buteyko-Methode" |
| Rita Fasel | „Die Spuren der Seele" |
| Gopal Norbert Klein | „Der Vagus-Schlüssel zur Traumaheilung" |
| Charles F. Haane | „Die erstaunlichen Geheimnisse der Yogis" |
| Verena König | „Bin ich traumatisiert?" |
| M. B. Rosenberg | „Nonviolent Communication" |

## Offers

1:1 Coaching
Masterclass
Weekends
Travelling
Training

**www.sanajer.ch**
*ckoller@sanajer.ch*

Register and get free access
to the colour illustrations.

## Imprint

© Christina Koller
1st edition June 2024 – Corrected 20 August 2024
VAGUS VERLAG, Switzerland
ISBN 978-3-9526041-2-0
Cover & graphic design Tatis Design Keller
Production: Libri Plureos GmbH, Friedensallee 273, 22763 Hamburg

**Photos**
Katja Meuli · cover, back cover, pages 8, 84

**Illustrations**
Tasnia Tarrana · pages 30, 31, 32, 39, 40, 53, 57
Tatis Design Keller · the wave